The Infertility Diaries

Inside the crazy, heartbreaking world of infertility told by
a highly emotional infertility survivor who swears she nearly lost her
mind more than once during her years of suffering with infertility.

Other Books by the Author:

Dancing Your Way to Fertility:
The Turning 40 Portrait
Early Morning Coffee
Tree House Cupcake Girls
Your Perfect Wedding
Diary in the Bed
Izzy and the Ice Skating Bakery
Stop Bullying Forever
Tonight at the Fire pit
The Amber Series
The Sammy Series
The Hope Chest
Its Not Your Fault Adam
Cat Tales: My Family and The Cats We Have Loved
Ask The Love Lady
Transference
Sarah and The Sunrock
Sunday at Grandma's
Sunday With Uncle Charlie
Tonight at Salisbury Beach

Visit www.paulafuocodavis.com to learn more!

The Infertility Diaries
Paula Fuoco Davis
PaulaMediaandEntertainment.com, Nashua, NH
ISBN: 0-9971459-1-9
978-0-997145-1-5
Edition Notice
Date of Publication: September 27, 2016
Number of Printings: First printing
Year of publication: 2016

This book is a combination of facts about Paula Fuoco Davis' fertility journey based on her memory, to the best of her ability. Names, dates, places, events may have been changed or altered. The reader should consider this book a work of literature. All statements, memories, descriptions, conversations in this book are the opinion only of the author. It is a work of literature and some of the conversations, quoted dialogue, experiences, statements, opinions, emotions expressed may be works of fiction. Some of the incidents and statements may be imaginary in nature. Parts of this book are to be classified as fiction, created by imagination and not based strictly on history or fact.

By reading this book, you agree to comply with the following:

This book's author, publisher, its affiliates or employees are not to be held responsible for any inaccuracies, omissions, editorial errors or any consequences resulting from the information provided.

This book's author, publisher, its affiliates and employees are not to be held responsible for any inaccuracies, omissions, misquotations in the book, and it will be considered a work of fiction, a piece of literature and a story created by imagination, not based strictly on history or fact.

By continuing to read this book, you indicate acceptance of these terms. Those who do not accept these terms should not read, access, use, interact with, view or listen to this book.

The material within this book is not intended to be a definitive set of instructions. Readers who fail to consult with appropriate health authorities assume the risk of any injuries.

The author and publisher of this book are not responsible for errors or omissions or resulting injury from anything written in this book.

The entire content of this book is not intended as a substitute for a medical diagnosis or treatment by qualified medical professionals. Please consult your physician for personalized medical advice.

Always seek the advice of a qualified healthcare provider with any questions regarding a medical condition, diagnosis, or treatment.

Never disregard or delay seeking professional medical advice or treatment because of something you have read or seen in this book.

This book does not promise a cure for infertility, or any guarantee regarding fertility.

The author and publisher shall have no liability or responsibility to any person or entity regarding any loss or damage incurred, or alleged to have incurred, directly or indirectly, due to the material contained in this book. Before taking any supplements, foods, vitamins, herbs or any other food or substance mentioned in this book, consult your health care provider for a thorough evaluation. A qualified physician should make a decision regarding foods, vitamins, herbs and other items that can enter the body based on each person's medical history and current prescriptions.

Note: all who choose to read this book should consult a doctor before taking any of the advice, information, outlined in this book. Before taking any supplements, herbs, vitamins, foods discussed in this book, all readers should consult with a physician about how these may interact with any medications they are currently taking. This book, the author and publisher, in no way promises or guarantees any cure or remedy for infertility or any other reproductive problem or challenge.

The reader should seek advice from a medical professional and a mental health professional before attempting anything in the book.

This book is not intended to be a substitute for the medical advice of a licensed physician. The reader should consult with their doctor in any matters relating to his/her health.

The author and publisher expressly disclaim responsibility for any adverse effect that may result from the use or application of the information contained in this book.

As an express condition to reading this book, and associated products, you must agree to the following terms. If you disagree with any of these terms, please do not read this book.

All material in this book is provided for your information only and may not be construed as medical advice or instruction. No action or inaction should be taken based on the contents of this information. Instead, readers should consult appropriate health professionals on any matter relating to their health and well-being.

The information in this book does not and is not intended to replace professional medical or nutritional advice.

The information contained in this book should not be considered complete and does not cover all diseases, ailments, physical conditions or their treatment. It should not be used in place of a call or visit to a medical,health or other competent professional, who should be consulted beforeadopting any of the suggestions in this book or drawing inferences from it.

The information about drugs, herbs, vitamins, foods, drinks, and any other food sources contained in this book is general in nature.

They do not cover all possible uses, actions, precautions, side effects, or interactions of the medicines mentioned, nor is the information intended as medical advice for individual problems or for making an evaluation as to the risks and benefits of taking a particular drug, vitamin, herb, supplement, or food.

This book and the operator(s) of this site specifically disclaim all responsibility for any liability, loss or risk, personal or otherwise, which is incurred as a consequence, directly or indirectly, of the use and application of any of the material on this site.

If you do anything recommended in this book without the supervision of a licensed medical doctor, you do so at your own risk because the information, remedies or exercise in this book may not be U.S. Food and Drug Administration (FDA) approved.

The medical information in this book is provided "as is" without any representations or warranties, express or implied.

You must not rely on the information in this book as an alternative to medical advice from your doctor or other professional health care provider.

If you think you may be suffering from any medical condition or before starting any new treatment you should seek immediate medical attention. Proper medical attention should always be sought for specific ailments.

Never disregard professional medical advice, delay in seeking medical treatment or discontinue medical treatment due to information obtained in this book

Any information provided in this book is not intended to diagnose, treat or cure infertility or any other illness, disease or medical condition.

Books may be purchased by contacting the publisher and author at books@paulamediaandentertainment.com.

Books may be purchased in quantity and/or special sales by contacting the publisher, PaulaMediaandEntertainment.com or by email at books@paulamediaandentertainment.com.

Library of Congress Catalog Number:
ISBN:
1. Infertility 2. Fertility 3. Health

First Edition

This book is dedicated to my mother, Sarah Fuoco for being the best mother in the world.

My father, Joseph Fuoco, for being one of the kindest men I ever met.

My beautiful children, Amber and Sammy, who God sent as an answer to all my prayers.

Jehovah God, who gives the privilege of prayer and who is always there.

My best friend, Leah Page Mortimer, who walked with me and helped me every step of the way.

My husband, Christopher Davis, for being there and walking this hard road with me. You were brave and kind, a true hero, and without you, I would not have my kids.

Table of Contents

The Doctor Called My Eggs "Bottom of the Barrel" — 20
The Start of My Journey — 22
Adjusting To A New Way of Life — 24
The First Ultrasound — 26
I Have Polyps — 29
A Month Later — 30
Hard Time of Year — 31
A Few Days Later — 34
A Visit to the Nutritionist — 34
Shivering At Night — 35
Rocky and Me — 35
A Meeting with Dr. P — 39
First IUI — 40
Trying Clomid — 41
A Request — 42
Very, Very Sad — 42
Meeting With Dr. P — 43
Date of Surgery — 44
The Donut Incentive — 45
Teaching Experience — 46
A Door Opens... — 49
In A Waiting Mode — 51
A Wedding — 52
Visits to Dr. Kim — 52
June IUI — 53
A Moment In Song — 53
Needing Validation — 55
Waiting for An Answer — 58
Screaming In the Darkness — 58
The Next Day — 65
Weekend Away — 69
Lapascropy — 70
Day After Operation — 72
Hope Comes — 74
Long Week — 76
Conference With Dr. P — 77
Getting Ready for Next Cycle — 78

Shot Talk   79
Shot Night   82
Another Shot Night   84
Back to the Pool   84
Getting Ready   85
The Night Before The IUI   86
Day of IUI   87
In Waiting Mode   88
For The Love of My Mother   91
Friday Came   93
Friday Night Longing   95
News Arrives   98
The Answer Comes   99
Yes, Its True   103
I Am A Pregnant Lady   103
A Third Yes!   104
Being Pregnant!   106
It's A Girl!   106
My Routine   108
Fourth Month   109
Gray Day in Pregnancy   111
Beautiful April 10 Baby Shower   114
My Baby Is Born   116

Part II: Secondary Infertility   119
Baby Making With Husband Nowhere In Sight   121
Third Try and You're Out?   124
Starting Down IVF Road   126
Physical Manifestation of My Internal Self   126
First IVF   128
Oops! Pee Pee Problem   131
Try, Try Again   132
Getting Happier   134
Writing My Life Story and Seeing Patterns   136
First Homeopathy Appointment   137
Needing People To Talk To   138
NOT MUCH IMPROVEMENT! Are you kidding me?   140
Praying Hard   141
On Track Like Never Before   143

Does Loss of Authentic Personality Equal Loss of Fertility?   144
Second Homeopathic Treatment   146
My Diet Is Actually Working   147
Back To the Clinic   149

What My Subconscious Had To Say: 150
A Look At My Most Private Journals

Fibroid Operation   163
Day After Fibroid Operation   167
And A Fibroid Would Have Been So Easy....   168
Preparing For IVF   170
Imagine   171
Transition Time   172
The Second IVF Begins Now   173
Cousin Lori's Wedding and the IVF   175
9/11   177
9/12 Day of IVF   181
Tonight's Explosion   182
Red Alert   184
Worst News   187
Chemical Pregnancy Nightmare   189
Devastating Meeting   190
Jealous and Ashamed Of It   196
Fair Time   198
Phone Conference With New Doctor   200
Riding the See-Saw   201
A Ride to Maine with Leah   202
Getting Ready for the Next IVF   203
Preparing to Conceive   204
Sunday Retrieval   204
Day of Transfer   206
Worn Out and Tired   207
Praying and Waiting   207
I Am Pregnant   208
One Month Pregnant   209
April and Still Pregnant   210

Today's Main Theme: Fear   213
Wishing For Popcorn and Molasses   214
June: Feeling Overwhelmed   215
Last Day of June   215
18 Days To Go   216
Countdown To My Son   216
Two Hours To Take-Off   218
The Birth Of My Son   219
The Beginning: A New Journey Has Begun   225

A Bonus Excerpt from Dancing Your Way To Fertility
Infertility: A Training Ground for Motherhood?   230
12 Cleanses to Help Restore Your Fertility   232
How To Improve Your Egg Quality   235

The People In Your Journey and Some of the   236
Rude Comments You May Hear Along The Way

Letting Go of the Secret Thoughts and Hidden Beliefs That   238
Might Be Holding You Back From Getting Pregnant

50 Creative Projects To Help You Tap Into Your Fertility   243
Letters To Yourself   246

I suffered and cried, but in the end my dream came true.

I want the same to happen to you.

I tried to put in this book everything I wish someone told me, so my journey would not have been so painful, and maybe I would have been successful a little bit sooner.

I wish you all the success you deserve.

Acknowledgements

Dr. Robert Deutsch for all you did to help me through my journey, and for being in my opinion, one of the greatest chiropractors and doctors in the world.

The reproductive center I went to, including Christine, ultrasound technician, for patiently helping me through many difficult ultrasounds and most of all, for being patient and kind during that first ultrasound where I could have given up. Thank you also to Carol for always holding my hand and being such a great support during my IUIs.

Dr. Samuel Pang and Dr. Goldstein, for never calling my eggs bottom of the barrel, for being kind, always trying and helping me.
Leah Page Mortimer, again, for everything.

Peter Rockett, for being one of my best friends ever.

My grandmother, Maria Fuoco, for your good advice and being there the night I announced I was pregnant. I love and miss you always.

My parents, Joseph and Sarah Fuoco, again, for every everything.

Mary, the nurse, at Holy Family Hospital, who knelt beside me and asked if I wanted to pray, as I was preparing for the caesarean.

Dr. Michel Lirrette, truly the best OB/GYN in the world. There is no one else I would have wanted as my doctor.

To Cindy Michaud St. Laurent, and her children, for visiting me the day my daughter was born and being the best friend anyone could wish for. Since ninth grade you've walked beside me and I am eternally grateful for that.

Paula Fuoco Davis: has been a a writer since she was in fourth grade and her beloved teacher Mrs. Klein knelt down and told her 'you could be a writer' after writing an essay about water. For more than 30 years, she worked as a newspaper reporter and journalist for The Lawrence Eagle-Tribune, The Nashua Telegraph and New Hampshire magazine. She covered education, social issues and features. She founded and is editor of Commitment.com, an online site for women and authored more than 25 books. She is a survivor of infertility and wants others to have every single bit of information she didn't have.

The Doctor Called My Eggs "Bottom of the Barrel"

My doctor looked at me point blank and said without a trace of mercy that my eggs were "bottom of the barrel."

Bottom of the barrel... Her words rang in my head like a cruel pronouncement.

I was 37 years old and desperately wanted a second child. My doctor didn't believe I could have one.

I had been through this before. To have my daughter, I endured 10 IUIs, several operations and too many nights of crying to count.

So I left her office: desperate, heartbroken, and wildly, frantically panicked. The words 'your eggs are bottom of the barrel' kept repeating in my head. Despite everything I've gone through, I always had hope. My insides were screaming: 'I can't live with this.' I was so shaken, I could barely drive home. Her words nearly broke my will and spirit to try again.

For some reason, on the way home, I stopped at a natural foods market. Walking around the supermarket, amidst all the healthy foods and supplements, I began to question what the doctor told me. Was the poor quality of my eggs something that could be improved? Was I unhealthy on some undetectable level that was impacting my fertility? I went home and called my ever-wise mother. She gave me great advice: dump that doctor and try again.

I did exactly what Mom said. I decided I would do everything I could to restore and heal my fertility, and not be hindered by my age, regardless of what the doctor said.

Over time, I learned that there was hope for me and others like me—and just because a doctor says you can never get pregnant does not mean your body, if given the right elements, cannot heal from infertility.

My devastation and despair turned to determination, and everything I learned, I put in this book. As a newspaper reporter for more than 25 years, I utilized my skills as a journalist to get to the root of fertility problems, the physical and the emotional.

I am now also a fertility success certified life coach and I wrote about how I healed my body in my book "Dancing Your Way to Fertility" that is also available on Amazon.com. That book includes my story, along with The Ultimate Fertility Success Program which I believe is one of the most comprehensive body-mind makeover plans available to fertility patients today.

The Ultimate Fertility Success Program includes 12 cleanses that will detoxify your body and expand your fertility potential. It will also show you how to improve the quality of your eggs— something previously not thought possible—and balance your hormones.

In this book, The Infertility Diaries, I share my personal journey of battling infertility, a rotten opponent that needed to be knocked upside its head and kicked to the curb.

It wasn't easy and there were moments, as you will read, that nearly broke me.

That doctor who claimed my eggs were 'bottom of the barrel' was wrong. Less than a year later, I gave birth to my beautiful son.

Someday, I would like to send her a picture of my boy and write in blazing letters across the picture: "Is this what bottom of the barrel looks like?"

The Start of My Journey

Today is my first day of writing a journal on my road to victory over infertility. I am writing this for women like me who have been told that their eggs are too old, that our bodies are too old, weak, or damaged, that there is little hope. I am writing this book for women who feel that having a child is some type of impossible dream, that they are the victim of some pathologically cruel biological problem.

I am writing this book for women who, like me, dream of starting a family, but find the road long, cruel, uphill, and not always forgiving of slight mistakes and accumulated years.

I am 36 years old. Last week, a doctor that seemed very kind when I first met her told me that my eggs were the 'bottom of the barrel.' I have been seething with pain and engulfed in sadness ever since.

'Bottom of the barrel' the very image leaves me feeling hopeless. I cannot yell at her. I cannot criticize her. For if I do, the clinic may label me 'psychologically unfit' to undergo further infertility treatments. So I stay quiet. I watch my words. I must adhere to and accept as normal their warped and perverse idea that pulling hope away is truly in the best interest of the patient, when with all my heart I know that it is only hope and faith that will ultimately give me the baby I so desperately want. What kind of monsters are they? I so want to walk into that clinic, tell that monster doctor disguised as a kind, caring medical professional off, and never step foot in there again. But then what? I have no choice but to bite my tongue, and wait until it is my turn to walk in there with a beautiful baby and say, "hello, do you want to see what bottom of the barrel looks like?' That is when my victory will be complete.

For now, I wait and suffer and try to erase their hopeless images from my head.

In this book, I will recount my experience with infertility.

I will tell you now that this book will end with my successfully creating the family I dream of.

I say this with confidence, for I believe God created us with a body that can heal and thrive and grow past illness, and that doctors do not understand the miracle of faith and the miracle of hope.

And for that doctor who tried to destroy my hope, I dedicate this book to you and anyone else who believes in stomping on a women's hope.

I don't always believe in being realistic—in putting my faith in only what I can see. Sometimes holding on to a dream takes being strong enough to push aside the skeptics, the cynics, the naysayers and delving into the world of hope--a world that takes a lot of strength to hold on to when everything around you is crumbling.

I begin this day by swimming. I am trying to get as healthy as possible. In the world of infertility, at 36, I am labeled old, but I don't feel old. Well, yes, maybe I do feel old. Withered inside at times. I just went through a harrowing IVF that ended with my becoming pregnant, only to lose the baby within two weeks of conception.

Cruel. That is how I feel right now about the past two weeks: cruel. They dubbed this pregnancy a chemical pregnancy, relegating it to something that almost didn't happen, didn't really happen, never existed. Thus was taken my right to feel sad or mourn, as it wasn't a pregnancy and it wasn't a miscarriage, but it was in a way, or is it? Nothing...dismiss it...mourning stamped invalid.

Most of all, I dedicate this book to God, who is the strength of my life. Without the privilege of prayer, I could not endure the hell of infertility. When the load was too heavy, it was only through prayer to God that I kept one foot in front of the other and kept trying.

So together, I begin this journey with you, a fellow infertility victim and survivor. I pray that we all see victory, in whatever form we wish it to come. For those of you wanting a child, I pray for your victory.

For those of you who have come to the point that adoption is a joyful option, I pray for you. I pray that we all can have the families we want and deserve, for family is a blessing and a gift, and all women deserve to receive this treasure of security, companionship, love and purpose.

Adjusting To A New Way of Life

In many ways, starting infertility treatments is like starting a new life—one I wasn't exactly ready for. I tip toed into this process, rather than diving headfirst into it. When I first began, I didn't think a lot about what was happening—all I knew is I wanted a baby and I felt safe that I was in the hands of a reputable fertility clinic. I didn't analyze much or have a well thought-out strategy.

I suppose, looking back, my tip toe approach worked for me, but it was not one I had the luxury of staying with for very long.

I was not prepared for how demanding treatments can be...blood tests at 6 a.m., ultrasounds, more blood tests, shots every night. I was often late for my appointments. I had a hard time juggling my work schedule and the demands of the clinic. I had not yet altered my life enough to include fertility. It felt like an interruption I wasn't yet ready to surrender to.

I felt like the clinic was constantly calling me wanting something...another blood test, one more ultra-sound—didn't they realize that if went to the 6:30 a.m. ultrasound, I would be exhausted by the time I got out of work at 9 o'clock?

Surrender...that is the word that describes the process in many ways. Battling infertility takes battling, but it also takes surrender. For someone like me, I had to progress to the point where the requirements of the clinic had to take priority over my own exhaustion, work schedule, social life, or personal desires.

At a certain point, the only personal desire I had to pay attention to was my desire for a baby.

For the first six months, I was consistently late for most of my appointments. I sometimes didn't show up due to my work schedule or car problems. I did this so many times, I finally got called on the carpet by Dr. P.

"Are you ready for this?" he asked. He told me that if I continued to miss appointments or show up late, the clinic could not continue treating me.

Talk about a wake-up call.

Suddenly, I realized that I had to take this whole process very seriously and live up to whatever it was the clinic asked of me, even when it was hard. I could blow my opportunity to have what I most wanted due to my own irresponsible behavior.

I explained to Dr. P some of the problems caused by my work schedule, and a few car problems that caused me to miss appointments.

He understood, but made it clear that this type of behavior couldn't continue and was not acceptable.

If I wanted their help, I had to be responsible. If I wanted these treatments to work, I had to commit to doing whatever they asked. Whenever they wanted me there, I had to be there.

Looking back, I consider this the first step in my training for motherhood: being responsible isn't an option.

I walked out of that appointment somber and scared.

I wanted a baby, and I would have to put aside whatever was preventing me from getting to my appointments on time.

This was one of the many turning points in my treatment.

Dr. P was forcing me to make a choice: continue life as you know it, without 6 a.m. blood tests, or go through this painful, inconvenient, life-interrupting process in order to get what you want most.

I left knowing I had to change, and this was one of the many times my infertility treatments would push me in ways that I needed to be pushed in order to become the mother I wanted to be.

The First Ultrasound

When I started infertility treatments, there was one moment where I almost gave up before I even started and detonated my chances of having a baby.

Recalling that moment is very painful, because I was seconds away from running away and giving up before I even gave infertility treatments a chance.

I never liked pap smears or invasive procedures. I've done then before, reluctantly, but I can't say I ever felt entirely comfortable with them.

The first time I had to do an ultrasound at the clinic, I was hit with a wave of fear. I never had a vaginal ultrasound before, and suddenly, surrounded by medical personnel, I felt overwhelmed

"I can't do this. I need to leave," I told Christine, one of the ultrasound technicians.

My fight-or-flight response had kicked into high gear: I wanted to run, escape, get out of there.

My mind was on one track and that was: I want out of here. All the appointments, the driving, it was too much.

All I kept thinking as I lay on that table was: 'I can't do this. I just can't do this. Maybe it was a mistake coming here. I'll find another way to get pregnant.'

Everything in me wanted to jump up from that table and run, and if it wasn't for the patience of Christine, the ultrasound technician, I probably would have left the clinic that day, and maybe blown my opportunity to get help getting pregnant.

"I need to leave," I told repeated. "I can't do this."

"Yes, you can," she said gently, never making me feel pressured or forced in any way to continue with the procedure. "You can do this."

She tenderly talked me into feeling more comfortable, and with her patient loving support, I didn't runaway. I started to calm down and despite feeling scared, I was able to get through the ultrasound. Christine looked and spoke to me with such compassion and gentleness, that the hammering fear inside my brain stopped, and I regained a measure of safety.

There were many, many more ultrasounds after that. Many IUIs and other procedures that were invasive and painful, but with the help of Christine and other technicians, I successfully did each one and became more and more comfortable, to the point that eventually doing a vaginal ultrasound or any other test almost felt like nothing at all.

I shudder to think of what might had happened had Christine not chosen to be so kind and patient with me that day. Would I have continued at the clinic if Christine had lost her patience, or been more concerned with rushing to the next patient, and not taken the time and care to help me stay put and get that much needed ultrasound?

What if I had run out due to my overwhelming fear, would I have ever gone back to that clinic--or any clinic for that matter? Would I have given up on having children, thinking I wasn't strong enough or brave enough to go through infertility treatments?

I shudder at the possibility that maybe that day,my fear could have resulted in a life changing decision. Had I run out, because some fight-or-flight trigger had gone off inside me, maybe that would have been my last attempt to go through infertility treatments. Maybe I would have resigned myself to defeat, never knowing I had it in me to endure the many painful tests infertility treatment requires. I did not realize that proving I could go through this first test would pave the way for my successfully going through dozens and dozens of painful tests later on.

That day, Christine wasn't just an ultrasound technician, she also became my infertility hero. She didn't have to give so much or try so hard to help me.

She could have said to herself: this woman is way too scared and too paranoid to endure the trauma of all the tests she will have to endure. Why should I give myself so much extra work in trying to keep her here? Let her go. Let her deal with her problems somewhere else. She seems like a paranoid person and I have a long list of patients waiting for their ultrasounds who won't take so much time and won't be so slow. Instead, she cared enough to slow down and gently coach me. She didn't make me feel like a freak or flawed in any way. She didn't shame or embarrass me for my fear, or insinuate I was weak, ill, or crazy. She was respectful and kind, and gave me exactly what I needed to endure this first test.

That would not be the last time Christine helped me and it would begin a very special friendship that continued for the next four years.

I beg infertility clinics across the country to look closely at their support staff, assistants and technicians. Is their staff truly understanding and are they trained to deal with the anxieties that patients may experience during treatments? Does the support staff take the extra time when needed to help a fearful patient?

Are they taught that it is important to treat clients with patience because certain tests and procedures can ignite complex emotions in infertility patients? Does the staff actually care about the person enduring these tests--or are they just consumed with their own work load and agenda? Do they slow things down, if it means getting a woman over the first rough initial stages of infertility testing? When hiring, do they not only look at the technicial qualifications of their support staff, but also the emotional qualifications? Is the staff truly kind? Compassionate? Empathetic to what infertility can cause a woman to feel?

To work in this field, you not only have to be medically and technically astute, you need tolerance, patience and understanding of the emotional hurdles patients like me must conquer to walk down this path.

Throughout the years I dealt with Christine, she was always kind and never once did she make me feel like a fool for being so afraid. With her, I never felt judged or put down. She didn't dismiss me, pity me, or treat me like I was odd or overly flawed.

She never showed anger at me for creating more work for her. She was caring enough to take the extra time to go very slowly with me.

Do you know how much I respect and completely admire this woman? She is one of the bright and shining stars of the medical profession. She talked me through that first day, which allowed me to continue my infertility process. That first day, it could have all ended. I never again after that felt a desire to runaway and escape the clinic.

That day, I might have allowed my fear to halt the whole process, but thanks to Christine, I kept going and didn't give up.

If it had not been for Christine's extraordinary patience, understanding, and kindness, I don't know where I'd be today.

Thank God Christine was doing my ultrasound that day. Thank God the clinic I went to had the insight to hire someone like Christine.

Thank you Christine.

I Have Polyps

All the tests have yielded one explanation thus far for my not getting pregnant: I have a polyp on my left ovary.

This is good news—finally some type of answer.

Last night, I went to the clinic to have some type of thing put in my vagina to prepare me for the operation...but when they found out I had a bad flu, the whole procedure was cancelled and rescheduled. I feel a bit relieved.

A Month Later...

A month has passed, and I'm back to have this thing put in my vagina to prepare for tomorrow's polyp removal.

It is so uncomfortable. Actually it hurt really bad. Tonight, I laid in bed and Chris rubbed my back until I went to sleep. This is so uncomfortable and awlful.

The most upsetting part of this procedure is the idea of going under anesthesia. I almost didn't want the operation because the whole anesthesia thing is frightening to me. I probably drove everyone crazy today asking about a million questions about anesthesia and the dangers of it. I talked to the anesthesiologist and he explained that now they insert a tube in your throat so they always know whether you are breathing or not, when in times past, they didn't have that precaution. That eased my fears a lot, because I remember all the horror stories about people going under anesthesia and never coming out.

The procedure turned out not to be bad at all. When I woke up, I barely felt sore.

Actually, I felt pretty good after the operation, except it was extremely boring to lay in the ugly recovery room waiting to be sent home. The room was gray, with metal pipes on the ceiling, and it looked like something left over from World War II. When we got home, Leah was waiting to greet me.

I am excited because maybe that polyp was my trouble all along--the hidden reason I was not getting pregnant. Maybe I will get pregnant next month! Good thing I came to this clinic or I would have never known about this polyp. Next month I can start on a new cycle. Maybe pregnancy is close behind.

Hard Time of Year

It is the week of Christmas and reminders that I have no children in my life are everywhere I turn.

I have no one to buy toys for, no one to bundle up and take sledding, no one to make hot chocolate for. Everywhere I look, there are commercials with beautiful little girls in pink and white dresses marveling at some wonderful new doll their mother has bought them.

Seeing it dangled before me constantly, I feel far removed from this normal and beautiful part of life.

I go in the Disney store at the mall and I run out almost immediately. When do I get a child to buy toys for? A child to tell whimsical fairy tales to? When does the magic I am seeing and hearing about all the time get to be mine to enjoy?

This feeling culminated when we visited my parents a few days ago for dinner.

I went there feeling depressed. It is December, and I am not pregnant yet. I am surrounded and constantly assaulted by visions of big families with lots of children gathering together. I see these images and ask: will I ever have this or will I always be so alone in this world?

When we got to my parent's house, I was feeling sorry for myself. I couldn't help feeling that this dinner shouldn't be so small.

The feeling was so overwhelming that I made a decision that day: this will be the last December I ever experience without a child in my life. If I don't get pregnant soon, I am going to adopt.

I was feeling pretty down, so I escaped to the upstairs bedroom. My husband followed me and asked what was wrong. I started to cry. He held me, and I told him it hurts so much to not have a baby yet... to month after month not be pregnant.

Just then, my father knocks on the door and wants to know what is wrong. I tell him about how hard it is for me to have yet another December come and go without a child in my life. He looks at me, obviously a bit confused, and says, "Can't we just have a nice day? We don't want the day ruined."

That was it for me. I was feeling very depressed to begin with, but this was too much. I storm downstairs, shouting a few choice words about his insensitivity, and lock myself in the downstairs bathroom.

I was not coming out until dinner was over and it was time to go home!

At that moment, I was already struggling to fight off my extreme disappointment and I had no stomach for my father's inability to understand the validity of my pain. I felt safer in the bathroom than being with someone who didn't fully get how beaten down a woman can feel when she is ready to welcome new members into her family, and those new members are not arriving as expected.

My mother and husband tried to get me to come out and enjoy dinner, but I just couldn't. I felt ashamed…a total loser…angry..So, so angry. I just wanted to stay hidden.

Maybe this wasn't the most mature response or the most considerate action to take, since my mother worked hard to prepare a lovely meal, but lately my emotions have been building towards a boiling point and once heated, I am unable turn them back.

I have little tolerance for all the people who take my feelings about being childless so lightly.

It seems everywhere I go, no one understands how painful infertility is-- a raw, blistering, heated pain that never lets up.

I need at least my family to understand how bad this feels.

Today I desperately needed them to understand just how hard it is for another family dinner to arrive and still it is just my tiny little family with no children.

Why couldn't my Dad see how hurt I am? How alone I feel? How horrible it is to experience life without a baby to love, when it seems every other family is overflowing with new babies, new children, a never ending supply of new life?

Where are the children who are suppose to be running around our family dinner table? When does new life get to come into our family?

On TV, I am barraged with images of big loving families with lots of adorable little children sitting at long beautifully set tables. I need that in my life.

I live in a dead zone with everything so stagnant and unchanging.

I need new babies at our family dinner table. I don't want another family dinner with the same cast of characters.

Give me new life, give me babies.

I want my Dad and everyone else to know that I feel like the loneliest freak in the world because I am without children. I feel like life is passing by me. Somehow, along the way, I got on the wrong track and something I was suppose to have has been stolen away.

I hurt so much. It was impossible for me to come out of the bathroom and pretend everything is fine. Nothing is fine.

It felt a lot less painful to lock myself in the bathroom than experience another family dinner with no children.

Chris eats quickly, thanks my mother, and we leave.

A Few Days Later

Now that a few days have passed, I understand a bit more clearly where my father was coming from when he said 'can't we just have a nice day.' He was excited to have us over for a visit and he wanted enjoy a good time. No dramatics. Just a quiet enjoyable dinner with his family.

He probably doesn't understand what the big deal is about having kids, especially since he only had me and what I have been to him is mostly trouble and upset. It must be very difficult for a logical man like my father to have a daughter like me--dramatic, sensitive, super emotional, always ready to launch into an emotional tirade about this or that.

Normally, my father is an incredibly loving man, but perhaps this time, he just didn't feel like dealing with my issues (trust me, over the years I have had a lot of them.) Maybe for once he wanted things to be easy, pleasant, simple. I can't say I blame him. Easy, pleasant and simple are words that do not in any way describe me.

I know he meant no harm. Still..I'll get over it. He's my Dad. He calls and apologies. A very nice apology. I accept and we make up.

But I meant it when I said this will be the last December I ever experience without a child in my life.

A Visit to the Nutritionist

I decide to get an appointment with an iridologist/nutritionist in Maine. I want to compliment my infertility treatments with holistic medicine so I can get to the root of my problem.

The nutritionist/iridologist is named Sarah M. and she comes highly recommended. She spends almost three hours with me. She starts by analyzing my body through iridology, which is taking an x-ray of my eye and looking at what it tells about my body. She asks me lots of questions. I tell her that I have no energy. Sometimes, by 1 o'clock in the afternoon, even if I've done nothing all morning, I am exhausted and just want to watch TV in bed.

She recommends a large number of vitamins and herbs. Since I can only afford to buy about five bottles, I ask her what are the top five supplements I need. She said not to worry: my father had called ahead and offered to pay for everything. That's my Dad for you—always so generous and obviously very sorry that he hurt my feelings a few weeks ago. I was so surprised and relieved—now I could get all the vitamins and herbs I needed! It seems my liver, blood and colon all need cleansing. I went home with about 15 bottles. I didn't even want to look at the bill since I felt so guilty that my Dad was paying. I know he spent a lot.

Shivering At Night

It is now the third day on Sarah's program and every night, I shiver in bed for hours before falling asleep. I know all the herbs and vitamins are cleaning me out in some way, removing toxins from my body, but it still feels horrible.

Rocky and Me

My treatment is not progressing the way I would like. It is has been a year since I started infertility treatments, with still no results.

So... I am marching... marching around and around my living room, to the theme song "Rocky."

I am doing this to psyche myself up to ask my doctor, Dr. P to start doing IUI's each cycle.

Time is passing and I feel panicky that I need them to do something more to increase my chances of getting pregnant.

A few months ago, I was a lot more relaxed about this—but now I am wondering: why am I not pregnant yet even though I have been taking Clomid for almost four months and my polyp was removed? Why am I still not pregnant?

I am so worried that Dr. P is going to refuse my request.

I've heard of people being kept on the same medications, doing the same procedures, for years without result, and I don't want to fall into that trap. I need an IUI.

Medication alone won't get me pregnant.

What if he says no? What if he feels it is too soon to move on to another level of treatment?

I play the theme song to 'Rocky' almost everyday on the CD player in my living room. I love this song. The beat, the tempo, bring me up to a victorious place, where even a loser like me can win.

I kind of feel like I am Rocky right now.

I put on the CD and I start marching around: *trying hard now...trying hard now...I am trying hard now. Its so hard now...*The drums beat...the trumphets announce a person is trying harder than they ever dreamed they could....

Give me a chance, Dr. P. Please give me a chance.

Getting strong now...Moving on now...Getting strong now...and the music starts to sound hopeful..like this man/me can climb this mountain, scale the wall, hit this victory...

I listen to the song over and over again. I march around my living room, picturing my ovaries turning, a baby sliding out, Dr. P saying yes to my request.

I listen and I march around the living room, my own homemade motivation clinic.

I have to be strong...strong enough to ask...to demand...to push...The medicine is not enough...I need more assistance...

Will my insurance cover an IUI?

What if Dr. P thinks I don't need to do this?

What if he says no?

Trying hard now...

Then what...what are my chances then?

Getting strong now...getting strong now...

I feel like such a loser right now, a faceless,
anonymous zero, and he is the almighty and powerful doctor who has
the power to decide my future.

Come on try

I need an IUI...and he needs to okay it.

I march some more, around my couch, my coffee table, up and down the
living room, around the table one more time.

It is raining out. I feel ridiculous, but something inside me is changing.
I'm pumped! The music moves me. It gives me hope, makes me imagine
that like Rocky, a big zero like me can somehow end up a winner.

Getting strong now

I imagine my baby. I see my ovaries turning and babies coming out.

I march.

I let the beat of victory pulsate through my tired sad, body.

My baby, my baby, my baby...I am a warrior setting out to battle and the
music beats strong....

Come on try now...

The music is my coach.

Will I take the right turn in the road? Will I say the right words, act the right way, have the right insurance, to make Dr. P do this?

I march for strength. I march because I need to be stronger than the doctor. I march for power because I have to make him listen to me.

Flying high now

I listen over and over again to this song, knowing that it is up to me to start directing the course of my treatments.

If he says no, I have to fight for my rights.

If he says no, I have to convince him. Stomp, demand, shout if I have to.

I've sat passively by for too long and it is getting me nowhere.

I need an IUI: I know it, can feel it. I need advanced help.

What I am doing now is leading me nowhere.

I need them to time my cycles, do everything to up my chances. I need help.

The music plays on and I am reminded that Rocky wins.

The music plays on and I don't know the outcome for me.

A baby, a baby, a baby....

This is my training ground. I am gearing up for a hefty battle. I am beat up, bloodied, and not a reigning champ by any means.

Around and around my living room I go, marching, walking, imagining myself victorious--ha!

I pump myself up, imagine Dr. P saying yes and me getting what I want.

I picture my ovaries churning around and around, like the wheels in an old mill, and babies coming out.

I march some more.

My baby....There is a point in the song where the music gains momentum.. where you can actually feel the hero rising to the occasion, stepping towards the exact moment where victory and defeat split in a fork in the road, and somehow the right road is taken leading to victory.

Will I take the right turn in the road?

I see my ovaries turning, churning, children jumping out of them. I see children..holding hands with one another...

Come on fly now...flying high now...Come on, fly...Fly...Fly....

A Meeting with Dr. P

Chris and I enter Dr. P's office prepared for battle. I have typed out all my reasons for wanting an IUI. I speak very slowly and seriously, anticipating denial and objection. It takes oh, about three minutes, for Dr. P. to say yes, of course, moving on to IUI's is fine. He shakes our hands, thanks us, instructs me to call on Day One of my next cycle, and in five minutes, we are done.

We both leave feeling relieved. We actually laugh a bit, feeling slightly silly that we expected such objection from him. Obviously, asking for an IUI is no big deal. He instructs me to continue to take Clomid and call on day one of my next cycle.

First IUI

If I thought a lot of blood tests and ultrasounds were needed when I was on Clomid, an IUI demands more than I imagined. Although as time passes, I am slowly getting more and more okay with the new demands. I am feeling able to cope with whatever the clinic asks of me. I have finally got the reality in my head that if I want a baby, I have to do whatever it takes to heal and get pregnant.

We get to the clinic and Chris goes into a room alone to give his sperm sample while I read magazines in the waiting room. I thinking how separate my husband and I are at this time, when normally we would be together.

About a half hour later, I am escorted into a room for the IUI. I know that normally husbands are present during this procedure, but I asked that Chris not to be there during this time.
Sometimes during this process, I get angry at Chris for no reason at all, because it is easy to want to blame someone and put my anger on a target, and most often, my husband is my favorite target.

Sometimes, I find I all too easily to pin my stress, fear and anger on him—it is your fault, his fault, not my fault, and so during this procedure, I want to be clear of these negative emotions. With strangers, I will not get so emotional, won't give in to the anger so easily, will force myself to stay a bit more positive.

I am so nervous. A technician named Carol is there with a nurse named Melissa. They insert a speculum and screw it in tight. I am not accustomed to this. It hurts and makes me feel trapped. Carol sees my fear and asks if I want to hold her hand. I do and it does help. Carol talks to me. She asks me questions to distract me and somehow I get through it.

The nurse removes the speculum, and tries a smaller speculum so it won't hurt me so badly. I so appreciate her gentle and extra effort.

Knowing that now my cycles will be timed by the clinic and I will be doing IUI's exactly when my body is ready and fertile is a huge relief.

Pregnancy shouldn't be too far behind.

I return tomorrow for one more IUI. It won't be long now...

Trying Clomid

They have had me on Clomid for four cycles now, which because of the delays due to the polyp operation, and my needing to take a month off here and there inbetween cycles, seven months have passed. Seven long months...

The other day, Christine, the ultrasound technician, cued me into something I should have known: she told me that Clomid usually works in the first three cycles, and if it doesn't work by then, usually another medication is needed.

Thank you Christine.

And hello doctor: why didn't you bother to mention that to me?

This made me realize how little I know about these medications, and how if you leave your treatment in the hands of busy doctors, you might never know when precious time is being wasted.

It also made me realize how helpful it is to know a person like Christine who lets you in on the little 'secrets' of the infertility quest.

I'm pissed of right now. Why didn't they tell me this? Why are they wasting my time? I need to write my doctor a letter and request that we move on to the next level of medication. I also need to educate myself about the medications I am on. Sitting back and trusting the medical professionals isn't a great idea when everyone is so overworked and busy.

A Request

I know that something is wrong with me that the clinic is not catching. Month after month, it is the same thing. I do an IUI cycle and the answer turns out to be no. No, no, no. No pregnancy. No, no, no. Why is nothing working? I decided today I'm going to write a letter to Dr. P requesting they do a lapascropy to check for endometriosis.

Maybe I have that, and they are not catching it. I'll type the letter, let them know I have some of the symptoms of endometriosis, and force them to look. They are wasting time and I don't have time to waste. I'm taking this into my own hands. I also want a different medication. If Clomid should have worked by now, I need to move on to something stronger.

Very, Very Sad

It is June. One year and three months since I began infertility treatments. Such a long time and still no baby. I am sad. No, I am beyond sad--I am enraged, frustrated, full of yearning.

I am tired of yearning.

I long to hold hands with a baby...a baby that is mine.

I look at mothers in supermarkets, mothers who look angry, tired and annoyed at their rambunctious little brats and I think: God, why can't that be me? Why can't I be pushing around a cart full of loud, overtired, rambunctious children?

These mothers look so overworked, and yet they have no idea that I would do anything to have what they have.

These women look deceivingly ordinary in so many ways, and I think: why can't I have their ordinary life--the one that includes a grocery cart full of babies?

There is a woman I see occasionally who has four young children. She is beautiful and her children are lovely too.

When I saw her holding hands with one of her young sons the other day, I was struck with that image--the image of a woman holding hands with her son.

Hands to hold. I want little hands to hold.

When I see the little hands of a baby, I think: what in the world must it feel like to hold the little hands of a baby that you gave birth to? What I would give to hold such little hands, to know those hands were mine to hold, to know that those were the hands of my daughter or my son?

I am going to write Dr. P a letter to ask that he do a lapascropy to see if I have a problem with endometriosis. I hope he listens and does what I want. I have to word the letter in a way that will get him to do as I ask.

I need little hands to hold. Hands that are all mine. To all the women I see shopping in supermarkets, who see themselves as ordinary mothers, I say--you have everything I want and there is nothing ordinary about your role as the mother to those little humans who are driving you crazy.

Please God, give me a little human to tire me out. Please let me be an ordinary mother in a supermarket one day.

I can't imagine anything in this world more special or more fun than pushing around my babies at the supermarket. My happy-ever-after is so plain and ordinary, boring even, and yet it feels so hopelessly impossible and faraway.

Meeting with Dr. P

I met with Dr. P today and found out a few disturbing things.

One is that yes, he knew I should be moving on to a stronger medicine, but because I tend to get scared and stressed during the procedures, he didn't think I could handle moving on to shots. I want to scream at him!

Instead, I force myself to stay calm and I explain to him that the more time that passes, the less nervous I am during procedures.

He seems skeptical, but I continue talking calmly, stating that while I may seem nervous, that is just my style of coping—and that the moment I leave the clinic, I feel completely calm and back to normal (which is true. I expulse everything and then I'm over it. It could be called being Italian, but I don't say that because it may sound weird.) He agrees to do the lapascropy and will schedule it soon. After that is done, depending on the outcome of the surgery, we will move on to shots. I am now waiting for a surgery date.

Date of Surgery

The surgery is scheduled for July 6. Almost two months away. I wish it could have been sooner, but at least I feel like progress is being made. Maybe I do have endometriosis and they never caught it. Maybe it is the reason I am not pregnant yet. As I write that, some anger comes up…Do I have to direct their every step? It is aggravating to think that if I hadn't spoke up, Dr. P might have kept me on Clomid indefinitely, all the time knowing that if it hasn't worked by yet, it probably was never going to work.

I feel a bit ashamed too, that my behavior made them think I couldn't handle shots. I can handle shots…Hell, I can handle anything if it gets me a baby…why would they assume that just because I am verbal about my fear it means I can't handle it?

If I silently suffer, does that mean I am handling the stress better than someone who is verbal about their fear? That is the odd thing about the culture we live in---people that hide their pain are presumed to be a lot stronger than those who verbalize it, but in some cases, the person who holds it in might be a lot more stressed than someone like me who gets it out and then is over it. It is hard to explain that to someone who doesn't cope in the same way, however, so I won't even try.

The Donut Incentive

They have ordered some new tests. This morning I was scheduled for a test I am dreading. I am so afraid of this particular test.

I don't think I have it in me to do this test. The whole drive down to the clinic, anxiety rattled around my body. How in the world am I going to make myself go through this test?

Then I got an idea: on the way to the clinic, I went to a drive-through Dunkin Donuts and ordered two of my favorite chocolate frosted donuts.

I get to the clinic, sit in the waiting room holding my donut bag, and soon am called in for the test. The nurse leaves the room while I change. When she comes back in, I am lying on the table, dressed in a johnny, with the donut bag sitting on my stomach.

"What are the donuts for?" she asks, straining to act like no-big-deal-so-what-if-a-bag-of-donuts-is-sitting-on-a-patient, but since she's not a professional actress, her irritation comes shining through.

"They are my reward for going through this test," I said.

My logic here is this: if I can lay here, endure whatever I have to endure, all the while seeing and smelling these two donuts that I am going to eat the moment the test is done, the test won't feel so bad or be so hard to take.

Nothing is a better reward for me than chocolate donuts.

The doctor comes in, and very politely asks if I want to eat the donuts sitting on my stomach before they do the test.

Again, he is trying to be nice, but obviously is a bit confused by the presence of the donut bag on my stomach. The great efforts everyone went through to show respect to me, even though I obviously looked eccentric, was both hilarious and touching.

What a nice group of people at this clinic.

"No," I giggled. "I'll eat them later," and it felt good to laugh and see the humor in this whole situation.

They did the test, and all the time I kept focusing on was: if I can get through this test, I can eat my donuts. I tried to think of nothing else, not the pain, not the nurses, not anything but the reward coming: the donuts.

How I love chocolate donuts.

The test ended. Everyone left the room. Before I even changed out of the johnny, I devoured the donuts in about ten seconds.

Ah, the power of chocolate donuts.

Even the most unpleasant test was bearable because I had two grand and delicious donuts to look forward to. Maybe I'll try this again.

Teaching Experience

I have one more IUI before my surgery in July. How great it would be if I got pregnant this time and never had to go through the surgery at all. Today I taught a magazine writing class at the community college I attended in the early 1980s. Since I am a reporter, teaching writing is something I do occasionally.

Typically, I love teaching. I teach one-day classes on Saturdays. Sometimes I teach journalism, sometimes writing your family history, sometimes magazine writing. Usually, teaching these classes leaves me with a buzz, a thrill, a high almost.

When I teach, I am seventeen and in love, I am six and allowed to go on the merry-go-round one more time, I am 11 years old and sitting in my treehouse, I am 14 and someone (anyone) thinks I am pretty.

When I teach, the insecure, negative, self-hating part of me disappears and I emerge strong, confident, and full of possibilities.

The girl in college who wore a white cotton dress and truly believed that anything and everything was possible returns briefly for an encore.

When I teach, I realize that my true calling was not working as a newspaper reporter, but being in a classroom with students.

But today, my teaching experience was completely different than usual and left me feeling pretty hysterical. Here's why.

The class started out as usual.

First, I introduce myself, and then I call each student up to my desk to talk one-on-one about why they took the class and what they hope to learn from the class.

The students come to my desk one at a time and share their goals for the class.

Now it is the turn of the woman sitting in the front row who looks to be in her mid-30s. Immediately, I like her. She seems spunky.

Then she opened her mouth, "I'm here to write about my seven year hell with infertility."

Wham--I am in for quite a ride.

For the next seven hours, eight counting lunch, all I hear about is her horrible experience with infertility and how it DIDN'T work out.

Her voice and desire to share her story was louder and more fervent than any other person in class. She had enough anger and fury to dominate the entire class discussion.

"The clinic tricked me."

"I tried everything and it didn't work."

"I'm trying Reiki now, hoping maybe that will work."

"All my husband and I ever wanted was children."

Even during lunch, when I hoped for a break from hearing about her pain, which scarily mirrored my own, she sat with me outside on the picnic bench and continued her story.

I felt for this woman. At another time, the teacher part of me might have been glad she took my class in order to share her pain.

But the infertility patient part of me wanted to tell her to shut up.

I struggled all day to remain professional, calm and not interject with my own experiences with infertility....but inside I was screaming was IS THIS GOING TO BE IN SEVEN YEARS? Am I going to turn into her eventually? Will I try and try like she did and never get a baby?

Was her lot my lot?

No, no, no, I kept saying to myself. I won't make the same mistakes she made. I was going to a highly reputable clinic. I was already working on improving my overall health.

But still....I felt panicked and scared. Hearing her story just confirmed all my worst fears: that I could do infertility treatments year after year after year with no result.

All she ever wanted was a baby. All I ever wanted was a baby. Were we two peas in the same hopeless pod?

I hid my feelings all day, knowing it would open a can of worms if I told her I too was in the midst of fertility treatments.

But now back at home, I am burning with pain. Will this be me in seven years?

She reminded me yet again of the terrible statistic that not everyone who goes to a fertility clinic ends up with a baby.

I can't stand to hear these statistics. They make me crazy.

I can't go seven more years without a child in my life. I won't be her, because if I don't get pregnant in one year, I will adopt.

I will always and forever keep trying for my own biological baby, but I will adopt before I let seven years pass without a child in my life. Hell, if I end up with both an adopted baby and a biological baby, what an incredible blessing that would be.

Everywhere I turn right now, I feel I am confronted with one hopeless infertility story after another.

Throughout the class, her pain was raw and rageful in a way I clearly understood, but surely didn't want to see, hear or understand. Why did she have to take my class? Was I suppose to hear something she said?

Was I suppose to know that sometimes this doesn't work out?

God help this woman, God help me. Let us both get the babies we so desperately want.

A Door Opens...

Lately, I'm realizing that to get pregnant, I need to get as healthy as I can. When I first started infertility treatments, I thought that infertility medicine alone would do the trick. Then I thought doing an IUI would guarantee a baby.

Now, I am beginning to see that more is needed to make this all work.

Today at work, I started feeling so nervous and desperate that I prayed all day for answers. Every spare minute I could, I asked God to help me give my body whatever it needs to get pregnant. I prayed repeatedly that God would help me get as healthy as I can be.

I feel so afraid that even with everything I am doing, it won't work out.

After work, I went to pick up Chris at the salon where he works as a massage therapist on Saturday.

I've driven that road dozens of times before, so it was odd that today, I noticed a sign I never noticed before: 'Chinese Herbalist'.

Something in me felt compelled to stop. I had recently read that Chinese herbs are sometimes used to help prepare the body for pregnancy. Maybe it wasn't an accident that my eyes landed straight on that sign, especially since I prayed so hard this morning.

I had to stop and see what this herbalist had to say about my condition, especially since I still had a few hours before my husband got off work.

Dr. Myung Kim would turn out to be an answer to my prayer. He turned out to also be an acupuncturist, and while he did not want to sell me any herbs, he recommended acupuncture. I tried acupuncture before and believe in it strongly.

He read my pulse, and told me that I had a weak gallbladder channel. I made my first appointment. He has even written a book on acupuncture.

It turns out that he has a second one about 15 minutes from my home, which I don't think is an accident considering how much I prayed this morning.

Although I have driven down this road about 100 times in the past year, I noticed his storefront today for the first time. Acupuncture needs to be part of my treatment, I am sure of it.

In A Waiting Mode

Getting pregnant has overtaken my thoughts like never before.

When I started infertility treatments last year, I felt an easy confidence: of course I will get pregnant soon, I thought, I'm going to a clinic, taking medication, this is going to work out.

Now that time has passed and I'm still not pregnant, a lot of fear has set in. I worry pretty much all the time.

What if I'm one of those women for whom infertility treatments don't work? What if I try and try and never get pregnant?

My desire for a baby has reached a point where what I think about and talk about most of the time is having a child: will I have a child? Why am I not pregnant?

Thank God that at work, we are allowed to talk during the day. I work in member outreach at a PBS station in Boston, MA, where we call members for donations. It is a part-time job that allows me to get insurance for me and my husband, the pay isn't bad, and it isn't so stressful that it takes up all the time and space in my life. It is the perfect job for this time in my life right now.

The best part of the job are the wonderful people I have met, Judy and Chelsea. We all are very comfortable with one another, natural friends and we share a lot with each other.

Judy has four children, and like myself, she cherishes children.

One day, out of the blue, Judy looked over at me and said, "I picture you with a daughter with corkscrew curly hair."

Hope! My dear friend was giving me hope! She was sharing with me a positive vision for my future! I can't thank Judy enough for gifting me with these words...words that I desperately need to hear. Hope is what I'm hanging on to by a thread right now...Hope...from a dear friend...much appreciated.

A Wedding

Today Chris and I attended the wedding of an old family friend. It was a beautiful wedding, and in the midst of it, one of my cousins heard a rumor that I was pregnant.

"Paula, are you pregnant?" she asked with a big, excited smile.

"Yes," I answered, knowing fully well I wasn't pregnant, but just wanting to feel for one moment how it feels to say 'yes, I am pregnant'.
A second later, I told the truth: "No I'm not pregnant...but I could be."

"You are!" she said, as if she figured out a big secret and I realized I had gone too far.

"Well, I'm trying. I don't think I actually am right now," I said.

She smiled and walked away.

I felt like such a loser. All my cousins at this event have babies..had them pretty much without even thinking about it...What an idiot I am.

Visits to Dr. Kim

I have now started going to Dr. Kim for acupuncture every week. I realize that to get pregnant, I need to get my body healthy on a very deep level. I feel like I am stepping up like never before.

I would love to be pregnant this cycle—then I wouldn't have to go through the laparoscopy. I have an IUI next week, and maybe this time it will work.

How great would it be if it turned out I got pregnant on this time—then no surgery, no chance of endometriosis, no going under anesthesia.

That would be so easy...

June IUI

Today, my husband and I did the IUI. We were incredibly stressed. As we walked out of the clinic, down the long sidewalk to the parking lot, we started fighting. Literally we burst out into a fight the moment we left the clinic. Lately, we fight before, during and after most IUI's. The stress builds and builds and at a certain point, we end up attacking each other like two animals in a cage. I hate him on days like this. He hates me equally back. I need him to be safe, calm, sweet. Instead, he feels like the enemy. We walked down that sidewalk, bickering and bickering...and looking back, I'm not sure about what. I said something...he said something..I got annoyed at his tone..he got annoyed at my tone.

We are definitely not helpful to one another during these stressful times. This whole process has been tough on our relationship. Lately, I see him as the cause of my infertility. What if we are one of those couples who just don't mate very well naturally? What if my body doesn't like his sperm? Not the kindest thoughts, but having a child is such a priority to me, I can't help but analyze him this way. There is no softness between us during these times, when I know there should be softness, but there is only anger and more anger.

A Moment In Song

Something wildly odd and beautiful happened this afternoon in the parking lot at the supermarket. I was there to meet a friend for coffee, and arrived a little early. Stuck with about an hour to kill, I decided to just listen to the radio.

I started praying about having a baby, as I usually do whenever I have a spare moment.

While I was doing that, Will Smith's "Just The Two of Us" came on the radio. The song is a father singing to his son. The Dad gives his son advice about not swearing, remembering to say your prayers, and holding the door open for girls. I love this song, as you can feel the power of this father's love for his child.

As I listened to the song, a wave of joy came over me--like someday I would actually be able to sing this song to my child.

I imagined that on my child's wedding day, I would play this for him or her, and recount this moment in the parking lot where I was begging for his/her birth.

It wouldn't matter if my child was a boy or a girl--this song would still apply. "Just the Two of Us"--me and my child. I got so deeply into this vision, of me dancing and singing this song to my child at their wedding, that it began to feel completely real. Of course I will have a baby someday! No doubt..it will come to pass...

The song moved me to another time and place, and it felt so completely real, that it was as if it had already happened.

By the end of the song, I was on a wild high, visions of my child dancing in my head: their wedding, their birth, this song being our song. For a few minutes, I landed in such a place of hope.

A good place...

For those few minutes, all the desperation I usually feel was swept away by a tidal wave of faith and hope.

Do I dare think this song was maybe a kind of answer to my prayer?

For a few minutes even after the song ended, a feeling of certainty that I would have a child was mine, all mine.

My prayer, coupled with that song, brought me to a place of joy I haven't felt in a long time.

My child was real--our relationship was real--the future with my child in it all became real.

Could this be a signal? I can't imagine the fullness I will someday feel if there was a little person on this earth I could actually sing and dedicate this song to.

Needing Validation

Everywhere I go, everything I do, in every conversation I have, I am looking for validation that yes, I am someday going to have a baby. I search conversations for clues, for hope, for someone to say "yes you Paula are going to have a baby."

People don't realize how their subtle words and expressions tell me volumes about what they really think about my quest to have a baby. A slight hesitation, a barely detected pause, the way they might casually say having kids is really no big deal, can send me plunging into a wordless, motionless depression. I am sensitive to the little nuisances in conversation that indicate the person doesn't really think a baby will ever come to me. I see it in that sort of shrugging expression people give when we get on the subject.

I need people to believe in me. I need friends to come right out and say: 'Yes You Can and Will Have a Baby!"

I want people around me to have no qualms about saying the most optimistic thing they can imagine saying to me.

I am hurt by all the people who see me as yet another statistic who won't get pregnant. The other day I was at the doctor's office getting a blood test when I came across an article on infertility and all the article did was rant on and on about the low success rate of infertility patients.

Why did they have this article available to all of us right their in the waiting room, while we are trying so hard despite the odds to get pregnant? Was it there to taunt and torment us?

I don't want to hear those statistics! I am tired of people imagining me a failure before I am ready to see myself that way.

One day at work, out of the blue, my dear friend Judy looked over at me and said, "I picture you with a curly-haired little girl." Imagine...out of the clear blue, she gifted me with a miraculous picture of hope! Judy sees me with a curly-haired daughter!

Does she know how much hope her words gave me that day? Does she know that her words released me from my sadness that day? Does anyone know how good it feels to know that someone else on this earth actually believes in my ability to give birth?

Why aren't more people like Judy? Why do so many people find it easier to believe I will never have a baby?

Lately, some people look at me like a lost cause. I am so tired of people who feel the need to share with me story after story of this person or that person who never could have children. Do people want to see me fail? Do they feel more secure in sharing bad news with me? Have they seen so much failure and disappointment in their own lives and in other people's lives, that they no longer believe a person can want something very badly and actually get it?

I don't know why their opinion means so much to me. I shouldn't need their validation so much. I know I shouldn't care what other people think, but I do.
I care because deep down, I agree with them: I don't believe in myself either.

A part of me feels this journey is going to be like lots of the other journeys in my life: me digging and digging for something, trying and trying, only to end up nowhere, and all my effort for nothing.

There is a part of me that has long believed my lot in life was to work and work for things, and end up with nothing. A part of me feels very comfortable on this path right now--doing lots of things without great hope or belief of ever reaping any reward for my efforts.

Many times in my life, almost reaching my goal has felt almost enough for me.

But this time, it has to be different. 'Almost' having a baby, 'almost' being pregnant doesn't count. When I was younger, sometimes I was content with 'almost'.

I even found comfort in all the 'almost' in my life--I almost finished my book for young people when I was in my 20s, I almost had my children's book published, I 'almost' married a man I had adored for years.

Almost felt comfortable--like that was all I deserved. This time, 'almost' can't be good enough--because the reality is, when I am 80 years old, there will be no 'almost baby' sitting beside me. I can't 'almost' be a mother and 'almost' have a baby. This time, I have to go all the way.

God, I want a child so badly. I want to love a little person so much. Will I work and work for this and never see any results for all my efforts?

I need people to believe in me, because I don't believe in myself. I need people to help me silence all the voices in my head telling me this won't work out.

Sometimes, I don't think I am normal enough to have a baby, which is suppose to be the most normal thing in the world for a woman to do.

Getting pregnant and having a baby seem the natural right for other women--women who are better, stronger, more deserving than me.

I seem doomed not to have the ordinary things other women have. I'm not quite sure why, but I've long felt this. Things other women get easily and take for granted seem nearly impossible for me.

I wish I could say to everyone around me: please, tell me I am going to have a baby. Don't be afraid to be crazily-over-the-top-optimistic about my chances.

Don't feed me any more reality stories about friends who tried for years to get pregnant and failed. Don't--please, please don't--tell me that God might have other plans for me. I don't want other plans. I can't see why God wouldn't want me to have a baby. Please don't speak for God and please don't assume that He is always ready to deny me what I want. Believe in me. Hope with me. Kick the odds and the statistics out and see me giving birth. And please, don't tell me life can still be enjoyed without children.

For once, I wish people would err on the side of optimism. I want people to believe in me. Please everybody, tell me lies even. Even if you don't believe in my ability to have a child, lie to me and pretend you do. Tell me I am definitely going to get pregnant.

Waiting for An Answer

Of all the IUI's I've done since I started treatments, this is the one that I absolutely and completely wish would work. I have to face a surgery in a few weeks if this doesn't work out. I've been doing this a long time. I absolutely have to be pregnant. I've been going to acupuncture, taking lots of vitamins and I feel my body getting stronger. I am waiting for an answer: please, please, let this time be a yes.

Screaming in the Darkness

Today, it came. While I was at work. I had wanted so much...hoped so much...prayed so much...please God, let this be the month. Let this be the month I am pregnant. I especially wanted to be pregnant because then I would not have to have the laparoscopy next week. The idea of going under anesthesia scares me. I so wanted to be pregnant so I wouldn't have to go through this procedure. A procedure that yes, I asked for, but that I still desperately hoped I wouldn't end up needing.

Instead, I went to the bathroom about 1:30 and it was there.

Gushing, spewing and mocking me.

Blood, blood, blood.

My period had, without a doubt, or even a trace of hope, arrived.

I sat in the bathroom stall, feeling like a tiny bomb has just gone off inside me.

Destruction lives.

I have no pride left now that I see it there. I have nothing.

I return to the office and don't bother to hide my tears or my disappointment.

"What's wrong?" asks Kevin, a very kindly young co-worker who sits next to me.

"I just found out I'm not pregnant," I blurt out, knowing it was totally inappropriate to say this to a single 20something male co-worker, but not really caring.

You would think I would have some pride, stifle my feelings, shut my mouth, but I am so desperate, I cannot keep my pain locked up inside me.

I have no choice but to let my pain be seen, so somehow I won't feel so alone.

Too much pain to keep inside. I will explode if I don't let it leak out a bit.

"Don't worry. That's not a big deal. You'll get pregnant," said Kevin.

Somehow Kevin's naive words made me feel better--but not for long.

Inside, I feel I'm at the end of a bridge, nowhere left to go, but down. I have been doing IUI's for six months now, and still no baby. Still no baby! Still no baby! Still no baby!!! STILL NO BABY!!!! Why???? Why no baby? Where is my baby? Still no baby! No baby--ever? Is no baby ever coming to me? Why? Will it happen? Please, please, please! Now! When? Why? Will I be old and without a child? Will I? No, no, NOOOOOO! I can't!!!

My friend Chelsea, who is sweet, soulful, sensitive, tries to comfort me the rest of the afternoon. At one point during our conversation, she said, "Paula, for some women, getting pregnant comes easy, even without them trying. For you, it is a long and difficult road, but it doesn't mean you can't arrive at the same destination as those other women. At the end of the road, you can have the same thing these other women have, but your road is going to be a lot harder."

At that moment, Chelsea gave me the hope I needed. She somehow changed how I saw my infertility.

Her words did not totally remove my pain, but suddenly I saw my journey ahead differently. Yes, it was going to be a hard road for me and it wasn't fair that other women could get pregnant easily, sometimes even when they didn't want to. But just because my road was difficult didn't mean I couldn't ultimately arrive at the same destination as the most super-fertile woman.

Maybe my road is longer, harder, sadder, but at the end of the road, I could be holding the same prize as all the women who have no trouble getting pregnant at all.

For a few minutes, Chelsea's words gave me a feeling of control and hope.

A new vision of my infertility entered my head: I saw myself walking on a dusty, dirty, rocky road. Big boulders everywhere. I had a hard road to walk, a walk where I get very dirty and tired. But at the end of the road, I see myself joining a group of happy women holding babies. They arrived there via a different road, a nicer smoothly paved road. But, at the end of the road, we all arrive at the same place and we are all holding our babies and we are all happy. Suddenly, my hard walk doesn't seem impossibly hard.

"Tonight, have a cup of tea or some soup. Something warm will make you feel better," Chelsea said.

Chelsea and I leave work at the same time. I thank her for all her kindness. She is a beautiful friend.

It is a hot June day, and on hot days, I feel worse emotionally than I do on cold days. Something about the heat makes my emotions boil over, whereas in the winter, my feelings can safely hide in the cold darkness. Right now, the summer sunshine feels like it is a mocking magnifying glass all over on my negative emotions.

I get in my car and drive home.

At work, surrounded by friends like Chelsea and Kevin, I feel supported, wrapped in the safe, warm blanket of a tribe. As crazy as I felt at work, I feel worse when I leave. The drive home magnifies my frustration.

Traffic.. heat.. trapped..going nowhere, my anger and fury heating up, so much so that by the time I get home, I am an inferno, a raging woman, entangled in frustration. In my heart, a raging fear that perhaps I will never have my own baby to love.

Chelsea's words provided me comfort, but now I am back to feeling cheated and desperate. I have hit an all-time low and every emotion inside me is roaring to be heard. Why did it have to be no this month? Couldn't for once things been easy for me? For once, couldn't this have been a yes?

The laparoscopy next week unnerves me, and I don't want to go through with it.

For once, just once, I wanted it all to work out in my favor.

My husband was sitting in the kitchen when I got home. I hate him right now. I truly hate him. I actually completely hate him. It is his fault I am not pregnant.

His sperm is no good, I just know it. If I had married someone else, with different genes and different sperm, I would be pregnant right now. I tell him this. I tell him how it is his fault I am not pregnant, and instead of being nice to me and accepting the blame and promising to do everything possible to fix his defective sperm, he gets angry, cold and defensive. He is not at all sorry that this is all the fault of his weird genes and his weak sperm.

We start to fight. It is dark now. We are upstairs in our bedroom. I need him to be nice, to hold me, to comfort me, but he doesn't do that. He won't do that. He is mean. I feel so crazy. I want a baby, I need a baby. I need him to listen, to understand, to be as comforting and nice as Chelsea was. He's never nice. He never helps me. He is never there when I need him. Can't he see how sad I am? Doesn't he care?

Why is he so mad? Why doesn't he hold me, comfort me, do something to make me feel like we will have a baby someday? He doesn't care, he doesn't try, he's never done the work needed to make this happen. It is always me doing everything. Me! Always me!

I can't stand it anymore! I can't stand him! I can't stand his stubbornness, his stupidity! I start crying.

I jump out of bed, grab a pillow and hit the bed. He is mean!! I hate him! I hate trying to have a baby with him!

"Do you think I will ever have a baby?" I ask pleadingly.

"I don't know," he shrugs. "Probably."

"Why do you say it like that?" I push. "You don't think I will ever have a baby do you?"

"Yah, you probably will," he says blankly.

"A girl? Do you think I'll have a girl? Or a boy? I want a girl first. What do you think?" I am pushing and pushing, feeling angrier and crazier by the minute. He says nothing.

For some reason, I have to know what he thinks. I persist, "Do you think I'll ever have a daughter?"

I ask this, because more than anything in this world, I want a daughter. A daughter...could you imagine the joy of having a daughter?

He answers: "Probably not. You'll probably never get the daughter you want because God hates you. He'll probably give you a son first, if you even get a baby."

Its all over now. I go crazy, ballistic, mad. His cruelty! At my lowest point! I have nothing left to hold on to now. I start throwing things around the bedroom. I knock over the VCR. I am going to kill him. He said out loud every fear that secretly lives inside me.

I am going to kill myself and him. I scream and I scream and I scream and I don't care if my neighbors hear me.

I scream so loud, I have lost my mind. I don't care. I am going to destroy him. I am married to a monster, an unfeeling monster.

My husband, who is suppose to be my support, telling me that God will never give me the daughter I want! How could he!!!!

This is too much, too horrible. I hate him with such intensity, I can barely... I scream again! I pick up all the books on my nightstand and I throw them.

How dare he intrude on my belief that God is going to help me! How dare he invade my brain and try to tear apart my one thread of hope that God is on my side.

Oh God, he is right. HE IS RIGHT! I'm not a good person. I am not good enough for God to help me get a baby. God hates me. He said out loud everything I've always feared, but secretly hoped wasn't true. What if I am not good enough for God to help me get a baby? What if God is punishing me, and will continue to punish me by not giving me a baby? What if God never gives me the daughter?

He knows--my horrible husband knows that the universe would never help a jerk like me.

I am helpless...how dare he steal my faith, my belief that God wants me to be happy and have a baby...how dare he! But... he is right, he is saying the truth: I am a bad person, and bad people don't get what they want.

I cry. I wail. I scream. Nothing but sadness and anger are running through my veins. I am forbidden every good thing in this world. I have no one, nowhere to turn. I am trapped.

It is dark. So dark. I see myself standing by the bed. I am so sad, so enraged. I scream so loud I know the neighbors can hear me. I wish I cared. I don't care. I howl in the night. I howl and I howl, because without God on my side, I cannot dare to ever hope to win this battle.

The night goes on and on and doesn't stop. It is all too much for me.

I can't feel these feelings, take this kind of suffering, to want a baby so badly, to need a child to love so much, and to be told by the person who is suppose to be your life partner that you will probably never get this baby, it is too much for me. The worst part is, he is probably right.

The pain is intense, the longing, looking at my life ahead as blank and lonely, to picture myself 70 or 80 and never having children, to always looking at other people with kids and envying them, wanting so much to love someone this way, and not having it.

The image of myself as old, alone, and hating what my life has become looms stark in my imagination. I get more support at work than in my own home. The night goes on. It never ends. This hell, my hell, never ends.

I am alone in the darkness, in the darkest night, and I am not good enough for anything normal in this world. He took away the only thing sustaining me. How dare he?

He is right! He is right...God hates me.

 I can't stop screaming!

Rage is pouring out of me. God hates me!

GOD HATES ME! I prayed and I prayed and I believed, and now I know I'm not good enough for God to help.

I have had sad horrible nights in my life before, but never have I lived a night with such a dark dead end, with no one to turn to and nowhere to go. A like this night that seems to never end. I scream and I scream and I scream. I don't stop screaming, because without God's help, I won't have a chance of this dream coming true.

It is dark and I scream some more. No where to go. No where to go.

At some point, I stop screaming, crawl back into bed, and fall asleep.

To this day, when I'm feeling sad, I remember Chelsea's words and I drink some tea or make some soup. But on that hot July day, I was at my wit's end. I didn't have any hope left inside of me

The Next Day

I woke up this morning raw, angry, stewing in last night's sadness, still feeling the sting of the fight...

My husband and I don't say much too each other. We are all fought out. Nothing left, not even anger to pass to each other. We mumble a few words, apologies, I'm-sorry/I'm sorry too.

Neither one of us are truly the monsters we were last night.

What reaction did I expect from him anyways—after I came home attacking his sperm? Did I expect warmth and kindness after I insulted him? What is wrong with me? Why did I think I could be so mean and disrespectful, and somehow get kindness and tenderness in return?

There is a knock at our door. It is our neighbor Richard, whose condo is attached to ours. He heard all the screaming and wants to know what happened last night. This doesn't feel like an intrusion to us. Our friendship with Richard is open this way: we are neighbors who watch over and take care of each other, and so it is normal that he wants to know what's up. He said his wife thought Chris was hitting me and she wanted him to come over and break up the fight. "I don't like to interfere between husband and wife," he said. "But we were worried." I assured him that Chris didn't hit me, and explained that I was screaming because I was sad over not being pregnant. Richard eyes us, like he doesn't quite believe our story. He is protective of both of us, and we thank him for stopping by.

His visit lightens things between us for a few minutes. His concern is endearing.

Today is Friday. We are suppose to be leaving for a weekend away to Deerfield, Massachusetts with my parents before my surgery on Tuesday. I've accepted that I have to go through this surgery. There will be no last minute surprises saving me from it.

We pack for the weekend trip and head up to my parent's house. We don't talk much on the way there. I feel too exhausted to talk.
I don't know if it because of my period or what, but by the time we get there, my stomach is hurting badly and I feel nauseous.

I lay down at my parents house for awhile, waiting for them to finish packing, and start to feel better, but that reprieve doesn't last long. "Time to leave," my father announces, and we head to the car for our drive to western, Massachusetts.

The back roads are twisty and winding and I feel so nauseous. I ask my husband to please stop the car so I can get some relief. He stops and I tumble out of the car, onto the lawn of a beautiful farmhouse and I vomit, right there on their front lawn. The grass feels so good, I just lay there for awhile, too sick to care.

We continue this way for the rest of the ride down...driving about 10 minutes..my stomach not being able to take it...my husband stopping and me crawling out of the car to vomit. I don't know now how many times he stopped, or how many times I ended up vomiting on someone's front lawn.

Finally, we get to the Main Street area of some sort of sad little run-down town, and my husband pulls into a donut shop that looks like it has seen better days.

At this point, I couldn't stand anymore: the stomach pain, the recurring thought that I will never get pregnant, was like a punch to the gut over and over again. My parents and husband go into the donut shop, but I sit on the front steps of the sad little donut shop and I begin to cry... loudly, and in a way I have never cried in public before.

I hear the song playing inside the donut shop "NECCO Beach" and I cry even louder because I went to a college with the initials NECC that everyone called NECCO, and it was a song popular when I was in college. When I think back to that time in my life, all I remember is sunshine and me wearing a white cotton dress, feeling like life was wonderful and every dream I had was absolutely within my reach.

The song makes me sob almost uncontrollably, because I am so far from being that happy girl in the white dress. Here, at this dirty old donut shop, 40 pounds overweight and powerless to have the baby I so want, is who I am now. Hearing that song from my college days seemed like a cruel mockery. I miss my friends from college, especially the ones from WRAZ, the college radio station. They were like a second family to me, and right now, I would give anything to have a place to go where people would accept me like they did. Remembering that feeling of walking into the radio station, filled with friends, was making me feel hysterical and making my stomach pains worse. Why am I not getting pregnant? I don't care anymore who is looking at me, which oddly in this town, no one seems to be doing. No one even seems to notice me crying. People walk by me like they've seen women crying desperately here many, many times before...just a standard for this run-down place. Is there so much sadness in this town that it is normal for a grown women to sit on the steps, clutching her stomach, crying? God knows how many people in this place have had their dreams shattered. Seeing me crying might just look like the norm here...just another loon with a broken heart.

The songs continues to play. Its not fair! I always thought I would have children young, but it doesn't seem like anything I envisioned for my life is coming true. Once, way back when, I naively wrote a list of the goals I wanted to reach by the time I was 30: I wanted to have two children and have won a Pulitzer Prize. Ha! What a complete laugh that turned out to be!

My life turned out to be one heartbreak after another. I feel crazy inside when I think about it.

So much pain bubbling up inside of me. I long for a child's gentle, soft magic in my life...a little person to love, a love that has nothing to do with romantic love or adult love.

The song continues to play, which makes it all the worse. What happened since college that led me to this moment? Why am I in this place? I can't walk through my life without children. It isn't what I imagined for my life. I always pictured and assumed that my life would include children.

I refuse to stuff it all down anymore. I can do nothing but surrender to my pain at this moment.

My mother, who is probably the only person in this world who actually loves me, tries to get me to come inside. I wish I could be alone with her right now. I feel badly that she has to see me, her daughter, like this, but I feel so tired inside from this quest to have a baby, that I can't stop this gush of despair anymore. My husband is trying to be nice to make up for last night, but I hate him right now and I don't want his kindness.

I finally go inside and lay down in a booth. My husband and father are sitting down, eating donuts like nothing is wrong. They try to cheer me up, the way a negligent dog owner would cheer up a not-so-beloved pain- in- the ass dog. I eat three chocolate donuts. They make me feel better. After awhile, we get back in the car to go to the hotel.

Finally, we arrive at our hotel. Once we check in, I ask for some time alone with my mother. My husband obliges, and goes to my father's room.

My mother comes in and sits on the bed next to me. Talking to my mother, as always, makes me feel better. My mother has a beautiful way of imparting hope, faith and confidence during life's darkest moments. She loves me, understands me like no one else, and says what I need to hear: yes, you will have a baby, she says with confidence.
Even though I know she is probably just saying what she knows I want to hear, her words give me a sense of peace. I relax for the first time in days. The movie "Titanic" is on a cable station. I loved that movie, saw it three times. We stop talking for awhile and just watch the movie.

When it ends, I thank my Mom and tell her I am ready to sleep. I am washed out from the nightmare of the past few days. On Tuesday, I am facing an operation that probably won't change anything at all.
But what choice do I have? Giving up is not an option. I can't live in a world without kids. If no children come to me, I will find a way to adopt. I am desperate to love a child.. to care for a child. I am tired of running around, looking to belong somewhere, when belonging never comes in any permanent form. But what if a baby never comes?

What if my life is spent searching? What if I end up being that sad girl on the steps of a dingy old donut shop longing for babies that never come?

I can't bear this. Sleep is a relief.

Weekend Away

This morning, I woke up feeling a bit calmer, washed out from the intense drama of the past few days. We went to breakfast at a nearby hotel this morning. It was delicious. Juice, toast, fruit. I'm trying to eat better (only ate one tiny piece of bacon). I'm beginning to feel a little better about my upcoming operation. I know I have to get it. There is no way around it--the operation will be in three days.

My weekend here in Deerfield turn out to be exactly what I needed: country, quiet, rural, green pastures and Main Streets full of houses with front porches. I wish I could live here...wish I could experience this type of peace in my life. We visit the Yankee Candle Factory, go out to dinner at an Italian restaurant, eat breakfast at a little diner. This is so good for me. I can't imagine what the operation is going to be like. I am scared, but less scared than I was a few days ago. I have no choice but to go ahead and do it. What if I have endometriosis and no one is catching it? What if it is the reason I'm not getting pregnant? Maybe this is the answer to my problem. We drive around a lot. I sit in the back seat, quietly enjoying the scenery of the beautiful mountains, the hills, greenery everywhere. This is exactly the type of landscape I enjoy. I wish I could sink into this landscape and stay forever. Let time stand still. How I wish my baby was here with me.

Will that baby ever come? If I let myself stay on that thought, craziness rises up within me again. But at least my rage and sadness has calmed a bit, and I'm beginning to accept what is going to happen on Tuesday.

Lapascropy

Today, July 5, was my laparoscopy. After the weekend away, I felt a little more ready for it.

I went in expecting it wouldn't be a big deal. I thought that maybe all my fears about the operation was for nothing—that the laparoscopy would end up being a lot like the operation to remove my polyps... a few hours later, I was back home, chomping down dinner and feeling fine.

Once I arrived at the hospital, I went to the outpatient area. Everyone was so nice, from the nurses to the young man who wheeled me to the operating room.

Right before I went in, I asked my doctor: Is everything going to be all right? and being the realist he is, he said, "There are no guarantees."

I prayed a lot. I prayed I would make it through the operation. I prayed, prayed, prayed. If this would bring me a step closer to having my baby, then it was worth it.

A few hours later, I wake up in a small gray recovery room, a curtain pulled around my bed. I have never felt such physical pain in my life. I am not sure what the pain is...

I ask if my husband could come see me. Forty minutes pass.
Finally, I'm sent to the recovery area.

My husband comes in. Oh God, it is so good to see him. The pain is so bad, I am crying. The nurse wants me to go to the bathroom--she says she cannot let me go home until I go to the bathroom. It hurts so much, I cannot imagine going to the bathroom.

Then, my husband kneels at the foot of my bed and starts to rub my feet.

He rubs and rubs them, trying to comfort me, and I think to myself that as long as I live, I will never forget the image of him, kneeling down, massaging my feet that day.

I just want to get out of there. I feel like the pain isn't going to stop if I stay here. I just want to go to my parent's house. All I want to do is leave, but because of a weird rule that you can't go home until you go to the bathroom, I'm forced to stay. The nurse is very kind. She sees that I can't stand being there. She keeps trying to call my doctor to ask my for permission to leave, but they can't find him.

I have never felt such pain. I can't even describe the pain. Finally, around 5 o'clock, they let me go. All I want to do is get to my parent's house.

Chris goes and gets the car and the nurse wheels me out. He jumps out of the car to help me. He is so kind. I feel horribly for how I've treated him the past few months.

I just want to be home, in my own bed.

Once we get on Route 128, the traffic is bumper-to-bumper, turtle to turtle, crawling down the highway, slowly and unbearably in the hot July sun. Obviously, I am not getting to my parent's house anytime soon. I am trapped on this forsaken highway. It is hot and we have no air conditioning in the car. I feel like vomiting.

The ride to my parent's home is slow. Slow, slow, slow, slow. The sun magnifies my pain, heats it up until it boils over, me in a steel cage, trapped by traffic every which way, the road feels longer and longer and longer, stretching out so far I feel like I will never get home. The window is down but no breeze blowing. It is such a long ride home.

I open the window and stick my head out.

I cannot stand it. I am going to throw myself out of the car. I tell my husband I am going to throw myself out of the car so an ambulance will have to come and rush me somewhere and I will have escaped this slow hell home.

Every mile down 128 feels like a victory, a step closer to
relief from my pain. Finally….(finally finally what seems like two hours
later) we reach Route 3.

The traffic is a bit better, but still so slow. My stomach hurts, everything
hurts. It is hot. Hot, hot, hot! I am trapped. I am an impatient child, who
cannot bear to wait a second longer. GET ME HOME! GET ME HOME!

Finally, we reach my parents house. I get out of the car as fast as I can,
run in the house straight up to bed. I don't even stop to talk to my
parents. I am a bit ashamed to be coming here to be cared for, but I can't
imagine going home and being alone when Chris is at work.

My mother brings me some tea, and oddly, instead of drinking it, I follow
my urge to put the tea bag on my stomach. I don't know why, but the hot
tea bag seems to immediately take away some of the pain. Heat. I
remember Chelsea's words about the hot tea. I ask for more hot tea
bags, and the heat seems to do the trick. I am starting to feel sleepy.

Perhaps I had been dreading this operation for a reason. What a painful
experience.

Day After Operation

I cannot believe what pain I'm still in. I wake up feeling terrible.

This is nothing like the polyp operation. This time the pain is sticking.

I am staying in my parent's bedroom. It is comforting here. Although,
this bedroom holds some difficult memories for me. About seven years
ago, when I was undergoing a severe depression, I got a terrible case of
strep throat. I neglected it for so long, that I ended up on the verge of
rheumatic fever, and the doctor said I should be quarantined until I was
better. So I left the apartment my roommate and I shared, and moved
home to recover. I was in bed for three weeks, but I can remember being
glad I was sick. Being sick was a relief, because I was in so much
emotional pain, that the illness afforded me the chance to zone out, do
nothing but watch daytime TV and eat my mother's fantastic Italian
cooking. It was a terribly low point in my life.

Being back in this room reminds me of that time. It isn't the bedroom of my childhood--that is the beautiful pink bedroom down the hall.

No, that bedroom holds happy memories for me. That was the bedroom of youth, hope, first love, ease, comfort, lots and lots of phone calls, and little sayings that hung on the wall like: *'when things go wrong like they sometimes will..when the road you are trudging seems all uphill...when the funds are low and the debt is high...when you want to smile, but have to sigh, when caring is pressing you down a bit, rest if you must, but just don't quit. Life is queer with its twists and turns, as all of us sometime learns, and one might have won about, would have won, had they stuck it out. "*

Wow--I still remember it. But that was a different bedroom, a different time. That bedroom seems too happy for me to recover in now. Besides, it has no TV and my parents were kind enough to turn over the bedroom with the TV for me to recover in, just as they did seven years ago when I came home to recover from strep throat.

A lot has happened since then. I actually fell in love with a good man and got married. But now, back in this bedroom, I'm reminded of all my failures, and here I am again failing to make the baby I desperately want. Why is everything about creating my own family so difficult for me?

I watch some TV today. It is a pathetic, but daytime TV is a mind-numbing comfort. It zones you out, tricks you into thinking you are engaging in some important learning experience, because a lot of the talk shows deal with the big deal issues women face, like rejection, poor self-esteem, and verbal abuse.

I brought up some stuff to work on my online magazine, Commitment, so I won't feel like I am just lying here going nowhere. Leah is going to come over later. Leah is such a comfort. My husband is back at work now, and he seems very faraway. I still can't believe how loving he was after the operation, how he massaged my feet...

I swear, that no matter what, the image of him at the foot of my bed, massaging my feet, when I was in so much pain, will forever stay with me.

The operation is over. Now what? One foot in front of the other. Inch by inch.

The words from the 'Don't Quit' poem that hanged in my childhood bedroom playing again in my head. Funny how things from childhood can be both a comfort and a foretelling.

Hope Comes

It has been three days since I arrived at my parent's house. I still feel very weak. I pray constantly. Having a baby feels like such a faraway dream, just another thing I'm shooting for that I probably won't get.

Prayer gives me hope, despite these negative feelings. If God could open the Red Sea, if He could save Daniel from the lion's den, if He could break down the walls of Jericho, I do believe He can help me. From this, I draw strength.

Today Leah and I went out to do a few errands. We ended up at Wal-Mart, where she needed to pick up some film for her upcoming cross-country trip.

While we were in the photo department, I spot a cute little photo album for babies that said on the cover, "Memories of First Summer." Leah caught me looking at it.

"Buy it," she said.

"Why?" I asked.

"Because next summer you will be using it," she said. Leah is always so encouraging, so positive. She is helping me believe that someday I will definitely have a baby.

"Paula, you need to buy this," she said again.

So, diving into her optimism, I bought it.

I will always be grateful to Leah for this moment, when she took my hand and helped me see a brighter moment ahead, when with my own eyes, it was hard to hope.

Leah and I have been here before.

About seven years ago, I was extremely depressed over a bad break-up, an engagement gone wrong. Leah and I were roommates, and one afternoon, we were sitting on the couch talking, surrounded by a bunch of lace and wedding veil that a friend of hers gave her after closing a wedding business. Suddenly, Leah walked over and placed the veil on me and insisted that I stand up and look in the mirror. "No," I kept refusing, wanting that veil off, because seeing myself ever getting married seemed impossible at that point. She persisted. Finally, I stood up and looked in the mirror, "I am going to see a happy ending for you," she said, with such positivity and love in her voice.

 I looked in the mirror and saw my eyes that looked dull, haunted, heartbroken, exhausted, "Sure. Nice thought," I thought to myself. "but no happy endings here."

Sure enough, Leah was right: a happy ending did come in the form of my husband.

Dare I believe her again? I left the store holding the book tightly in my hands.

Tonight, I put the little photo album on my nightstand. I am so afraid I will lose it, and that will be a sign that my baby's picture will never be in it.

I check and recheck that the album is still there several times before letting myself fall asleep.

Leah and I have always been each other's cheerleaders when it comes to reaching our dreams. I believe she really does believe I'll have a baby. Just the way she believed I would find love again way back then.

What better gift can a friend give? Then to bestow upon another hope, a sense of believing that the one thing truly wished for will actually come true.

So I have this photo album, but I don't feel fully convinced that I will ever get to use it. I lift my head off the pillow, one more time, to make sure it is still on the nightstand before heading off to sleep.

Long Week

This has been one long and tedious week. The pain from the lapascropy has continued much longer than I ever imagined.

I didn't feel much like talking this week. Between the pain, the fatigue, and my sadness, I prefer to be quiet right now. So unlike the me from the past, when all I wanted to do was talk.

This time, I feel myself sinking inward to deal with my emotions.

Most of the words coming towards me from the outside world, even from well-meaning people, ring with the tune of: "There goes Paula again, trying for something she will never get." I sometimes feel like they all know the end of my fertility story, and I am the only one stupid enough to believe this can actually work out.

I just can't hear words like, "maybe God doesn't want you to have a baby" or 'maybe you are meant to do something else" or "God knows what we can handle" or "you have to just accept what God gives you." Bah hum bug! That's what I say to all of them. I no longer will talk about this with anyone who even slightly tries to prepare me for failure. They all think I am going to fail, and if I listen to them, I will believe them and my body will never let me produce a baby.

So, for maybe the first time in my life, I don't want to share what I am going through with anyone. I watched a lot of TV this week, and I went on my father's computer about an hour a day to work on my online magazine I enjoy so much.

It is called Commitment and I have big dreams for that magazine.. All my big dreams. Sometimes I feel like I am digging and digging a hole that ultimately will go nowhere. For most of my life, there is something inside me that has always believed I should work and work and work, but ultimately get nowhere for all my effort.

A part of me still feels that way, and having a baby seems to fall into that category.

In a few days, I return home and start again on a new cycle. I've decided that if a baby is not here by December, I am going to look into adoption, while still trying for my own biological baby. I so much need a little person to love.

Conference With Dr. P

We met with Dr. P. today to discuss the results of the laparoscopy. I was surprised to hear that I do not have endometriosis. In fact, Dr. P says I was pretty "clean" as he put it. In a way, I am relieved, but in another way it hurts to think the entire operation was a waste. At least if I had endometriosis there would be an explanation as to why I am not getting pregnant.

Well, I did read once about a women who got pregnant after a laparoscopy because it cleared her fallopian tubes or something…so maybe it wasn't a total waste.

Anyways, I am moving past Clomid and on to more powerful medications in the form of shots. Dr. P. asks me again if I can handle the shots. He feels reluctant because of the hard time I've had with some of the tests in the past.

"Are you going to be able to do this?" he asks.

"YES YES YES" I wanted to scream. "GET ME THE SHOTS! I CAN TAKE THE SHOTS IF THEY WILL GIVE ME A BABY!"

My husband and I have to take a class on the shots. I'm nervous, but more than willing to do them.

Hell, if this is what I need, I wish they had moved me on to shots a long time ago. What my doctor, and most of the people here. don't realize is, while I may whine and whimper over my tests, I would do 1,000 shots if that is what it will take to get a baby.

What I want to say to Dr. P is: "just because I have a hard time with the tests, and I ask that someone hold my hand during the IUI's doesn't mean I can't endure more pain.

I'll take whatever, maybe whimpering and whining the whole time, but I'll take it, and continue more if that what I have to do.'

One thing this whole infertility mess has taught me is if you want something bad enough, you have to be willing to pay whatever price is asked. I read that in a self-help book recently--if you want something, you have to be willing to throw yourself over the bar, walk through the fire, in order to get what you want.

Would I walk through fire to have a baby? Yes, I would. I think I can honestly say I would do anything asked of me. So, yes Dr. P, I'm ready for the shots. All you can see is the whimpering me, but what you don't know is that I won't stop at anything.

 It is odd that if I was quiet and kept my fears locked up inside, maybe so much so that I might destroy myself, they would deem me better able to cope. Don't they understand that it is because I talk about my fears and ask for what I need that I can do this. Go figure.

We scheduled a date for class and get ready for the next cycle. I plan on doing everything I can to make this work.

Getting Ready for Next Cycle

I'm now focused on getting ready for the next IUI cycle.

 I've decided that I'll take a week off of work right after the IUI and stay with my parents at the beach.

Ever since I was 10 years old, my parents have rented at Salisbury Beach, an old-time honky-tonk beach to some, but to my family, the absolutely most beautiful beach in the world.

Maybe some rest and relaxation at the beach will help. I read a lot lately about how reduced stress levels increase the chances of getting pregnant. I'm skeptical, but willing to try it. My boss won't be thrilled. August is pledge month and they need as many callers as possible. I almost don't want the week off, because I like work and I hate displeasing my boss, but I have to put getting pregnant above anything else. I keep picturing myself 80 years old and it is doubtful my friends at work will be with me.

 So I'm putting in for the time off. I have to keep the big picture in my head.

Shot Talk

 Today, my husband attended a class on how to administer the shots. My husband tells me he is certain he can do this.

We start the shots tonight.

At work, I started feeling so anxious about the shots and what lay ahead of me: will they hurt? Can I handle it? How bad will it be?

I was getting so nervous, I started chatting about the shots today at work. Chatting and talking lightly, almost jovially about it, as if I was talking about an upcoming vacation, or a recent trip to the dentist.

That's how I cope--I open up, spill my guts to the world, make light of my sorrows publicly, put myself on display, like a joke or something, all in an effort to rally the troops around me.

To me, it is easier to open up than keep it inside and carry the burden alone.

Here at work, I feel safe, comfortable, at home and accepted by my work family, a group of people I've come to love, trust, and feel able to share my struggles. Inbetween our phone calls, we talk about everything, from high school crushes, best friends who ditched us, childhood bedrooms, favorite books, worst rejections, biggest disappointments, dolls that we lost, favorite foods, and songs from the 1970s that still make us cry.

I know infertility isn't a light hearted subject--certainly not fodder for slow work day chatter, but that's how I get through the days--talking so much everything starts to seem like no big deal even to myself.

The more I talk about it, the more minor it all seems. The more I hold it up to the light of day, the smaller it becomes. It cannot eat me alive if I spit it out for all to see. If I keep it in, make it too sacred to talk about, then it becomes something more than I can take.

The fact is, talking to my closest friends I've had for years is hard. They've seen me want things before—things that didn't work out. They also know the ugly truth that it ain't pretty when I'm devastated.

So when I voice my incessant longing for a child, they remember me broken, and they don't want to see that again--so they try to prepare and cushion me for disappointment.

I understand where they are coming from. but I can't bear that type of comfort right now. For me to someday give birth, I have to put aside every failure in my life, which have been many, and somehow believe this time will be different. I have to see myself as a person for whom a happy ending is possible.

So I talk to my new friends at work, friends who see a lighter, happier side of me, friends who can believe in my dream, because they do not fear so much for my failure.

Here in our cubicle-filled office with no windows to the outside world, I feel insulated from the realities of my life. I feel so cushioned here, that any sadness and heartbreak I've experienced in my life seems like just another dramatic or funny story to tell.

Suddenly things that shamed me seem like material for tomorrow's good story. I don't hate myself as much anymore, because when I share my stories, I see myself in a different way—I am funny, quirky, creative, original—what was all that self-hatred about? Even the saddest parts of my life don't seem as half as sad when I talk about them at work.

Yet, without knowing it today, I hit upon a subject that was difficult for one of my co-workers and friend. She pulled me into a side room to tell me that she was not at all happy about my chattering about the shots. It turns out, she has been going through infertility treatments for ten years, and the shots are very painful, hard to administer and she ended up never getting pregnant. She told me to ask my doctor about what was in the medication I'm taking, because it could cause cancer.

She had chosen to be very selective about whom she talked to about her infertility, and she didn't appreciate my talking so lightly about a very serious subject.

I feel ashamed, and then I wonder: what if she is right? What if my husband has trouble giving me the shots? What if I do all this and it doesn't work out? What if all this medicine gives me is cancer, instead of a baby?

I thank her, but in that moment, I have no choice but to blank out all the warnings. I want a baby so badly, I have no choice but to take some risks.

Whatever the medicine is, I need it, poison or not.

Why should I have to keep quiet about my infertility? I'm not a bad woman because my body isn't producing a baby. My friend, also, should not have had to feel ashamed about her infertility, as she is an awesome, amazing woman. Why can other people talk about their health challenges but infertility is something best to keep hushed up?

There is still so much shame tied up with this illness. Does infertility mark us as flawed? Bad woman having problems related to sex and marriage, inferior to those fertile lovelies who get pregnant without even trying?

Why are we seen as desperate if we say right out loud that we long for a baby and we are devastated because it isn't happening as fast or as naturally as we imagined? Is it because all things pertaining to motherhood and woman in general are disrespected?

There are all sorts of moral parables tied up in not getting pregnant--that God is denying you a baby, or that you are not up to the job of being a parent, or that you are suppose to adopt or that you are just not good enough to bear a child.

Tonight, my husband has to jab needles into my body. I'm almost too scared to go through with it. Just thinking about the shots makes everything in my life seem hard and heavy.

That's why I can't stay quiet --because once I stay quiet, it all becomes too horrible, too ugly, too awlful to endure. I need people to listen. By talking about it lightly, I am convincing myself that taking the shots is really no big deal.

So I will talk and chatter and make light of what I am facing in a few hours. I'm not ashamed of having a problem making a baby.

I don't need to hang my head in shame over this.

Shot Night

Tonight, for the first time, my husband administered the shots. All day long, I felt a heaviness hanging over me. At 2 p.m. it was five hours away. At 3 p.m. four hours away. At 4 p.m., three hours away.

Finally, it was 7 o'clock. My husband starts by opening the bottles to prepare the medication. I admire his bravery, as I watch him mix the medicines.

Then I sit down in the kitchen. I've learned a few tricks about taking tests:

1) Don't look. Keep your eyes shut. Seeing it only make the pain more intense.

2) Breath out, while blowing, blowing, blowing, kind of like as substitution.

3) Distract yourself with something fun, comforting or sweet.

4) Have a reward waiting.

Here's how I distracted myself tonight: I recently got a cookbook with recipes from bed and breakfast inns.

The book has a beautiful blue and white cover and it is all about cozy, comfortable, romantic places..the delightful stuff bed & breakfast inns are made of.

I opened the book and decide that while I am getting a shot, I will read a recipe--knowing that by the time I get to the end of the recipe, the shot will be over.

We're just about ready. I am praying every moment for the strength to endure this. My husband looks for a spot on my leg. I look away.
I open to a recipe and start reading. The book is comforting and I am transported to a beautiful place.

My husband jabs the needle into my leg, quickly, so quickly, I breath, breath, breath. I pray. I start reading a recipe, and it is over. I've reached the end of my recipe.

Then, like a spring day after a storm, a bit of alcohol to clean it, a bandage and I am free. Tomorrow, I will think about the next shot. But for tonight, it is over and done. It hurt, but not half as bad as I imagined.

Now I can just sit back and enjoy tonight.

Another Shot Night

I'm getting more comfortable with the actual shots, although in the hours leading up to them, I am overcome with a lot of anxiety and dread.

Tonight, some of Chris's friends came over and we went ahead with the shots, despite the fact that they were all standing two feet away in our living room.

Having a bunch of guys standing outside the kitchen, practically watching me get shots, brought an air of humor to this. These guys are mostly single, so completely out-of-touch with this type of stuff, and so it was funny to see them privy to what is normally such an intimate and hush-hush procedure.

They actually seemed scared in a way, and that made the whole thing all the more humorous to me.

Back to the Pool

In preparing for my next IUI, I am eager to start my morning swim routine. After reading about the link between stress and infertility, I realized that I needed to find a way to release my stress.
Since swimming has always relaxed me, and I chose swimming as one of the ways I am going to release the stress in my life.

At first, my husband was skeptical. "Are you really going to get up early every morning and go swimming before work?" he asked.

"Yeeees," I replied with great irritation. "Just watch me."

So every morning (well, almost every morning) between 5:30 and 6 o'clock, I wake up, creep quietly out of bed, put my towel in the bag, check to make sure I have my club ID, and then I head down to the door, hoping it won't wake my husband.

I like the whole rhythm of going for a swim in the early morning.

I like the way the sun cocks its head and shines that time of morning, as if to say hello and welcome to your day. I like the early morning drive, with so few cars on the road, lots good music on the radio, and the sense that by getting out the door early, I am part of the early mornings' rock and roll.

The first day I went to swim, I was terrified, like the shy awkward kid on the first day of junior high. There is always a moment of fear right before I go in the water: Can I actually do this? Actually go in the pool? What if the water is cold? What if the water is too cold for me to take? I throw my body in anyways, and it feels like a moment of triumph.

One day, something odd happened. I swam 40 minutes straight. Being 40 pounds overweight and out of shape, this was a lot longer than normal for me. Afterwards, I felt limp and floppy. When I got in the car to drive home, I suddenly burst out crying—but it was an odd type of crying, because I didn't feel any emotion. It was more of a physical releasing cry than an emotional cry. I wasn't thinking of anything particularly sad. It was as if my body was just releasing. I sat in my car, just crying and crying. By the time I got home, I had stopped crying and a crazy massive feeling of joy had overtook me. Joy as I went in the house! Joy as I ran up the stairs to my bedroom! Joy ! Joy! Joy!

Something bad left my body that day and it was replaced by a light-heartedness I had not felt in a long, long time.

My husband immediately noticed the change in me. "you seem so relaxed," he said.

When I swim, I am proving to myself that I can do what it takes to win this battle with infertility.

Getting Ready

I feel a momentum building towards the IUI coming up next week. I've gone to Dr. Kim for acupuncture treatments three times so far.

I know it is a lot, and that we can't really afford it, but I need to do everything up my chances.

I made Chris go twice, as it can't hurt if his body is operating better too. Between the swimming, acupuncture and eating better, I feel my health is changing I took next week off so I can stay with my parents at the beach. Doing the IUI and then having a week to relax at the beach should help this whole getting-pregnant-process. Lots of praying daily too.

The Night Before The IUI

It is Saturday and I'm here at the beach with my parents. They are renting a house for three weeks. It is the same beach we have stayed at since I was a kid and so my family has loads of wonderful memories tied up at this beach. Things have been going well in preparation for tomorrow's IUI. I feel oddly happy and optimistic even. I took the week out of work so I could stay here at the beach and rest after the IUI. The water, the sunshine, the chance to sit and do nothing, should up my chances of getting pregnant. I took the week off during my department's busiest time, but all my choices right now have to be for my baby. Work and everything else cannot matter right now.

Tonight, we are taking it easy. I had a nice meal. I ate lots of plums, because I've been reading about the blood type diet and plums are suppose to be good for O blood types.

All my hard work has paid off in one way so far: I feel much better than I used to feel.

I had three acupuncture treatments in the past six days, and I made Chris go twice. Even though we can't really afford it, I pushed Chris and begged for this. I know the more acupuncture I have, the better. It will clear my energy, enhance my life force, make me stronger. Dr. Kim is marvelous.

Tomorrow, a new life begins...it has to...I beg God for this.

Day of IUI

Today is Sunday, August 2. I felt happy on the ride to the clinic this morning, the sun shining with a big grin, and a week at the beach I love ahead of me. Thank God there was no traffic this morning.
Driving to the clinic is normally so hard, scary, stressful and frantic.

Today, on an early Sunday morning, a piece of cake. From the beach, we took a different route than we usually go and everything just felt easier, safer and more joyous than usual. No 128 traffic!

I did something a bit different than usual too--I brought along a bottle of red wine!

Last week at work, Judy told me she thought that a glass of wine can sometimes help a person relax and have a better chance of getting pregnant. I listened and decided I would drink some wine before the procedure.

Once we were inside the waiting room, I realized that I had forgotten the wine in the car.

"Go get it," I whispered to my husband.

"Really? You want it?" he hemmed and hawed.

'Yes, please," I said, feeling an urgency to try something different this time.

"You can't drink it here," he said.

"I'll go in the bathroom," I whispered.

Kooky, yes, but what the heck. I needed to relax.

He went to the car, came back in with the wine bottle hidden under his shirt. He passed it to me discreetly, I put it under my shirt, went into the bathroom, and slugged a bit down.

Well, at the very least, I immediately feel more relaxed—and it felt pretty good to do something so forbidden at the clinic.

My husband went first, as he always does, to give his sperm. I have no idea what this is like for him. We never talk about it.
A while later, they call me in. I hate the whole IUI process. I hate the speculum they put inside me, that is so tight when they screw it in. Every moment the speculum is inside me is difficult and painful, and when they finally start to unscrew it, a huge relief passes through me.

Thankfully, the nurses hold my hand and talk to me during the IUI. They ask me questions, like what movies I saw recently and what I do for work. They are so kind.

Today, the IUI is done by Melissa and it is quick. She always does a good job. Then, my husband comes in and I continue laying on the table. I put my legs high up in the air, against the wall, hoping this will help the sperm get to where it needs to go. I do this for 40 minutes, even though they say you can leave in 10 minutes. We decide to wait as long as we can. Give that sperm some help swimming up! Will it happen this time? Hope lives in my heart. I pray fervently, night and day, for my baby to come alive. Oh God, please. I know that the only hope I have is that God hears my prayer, and because of that hope, I do feel hope despite everything. Oh God, please.

We return to the beach, and enjoy a quiet evening sitting by the ocean. I eat lots of dark purple plums. Did the IUI work? Two weeks from now, we'll know the answer.

In Waiting Mode

Now that the IUI is done, I am in a waiting mode. It is very relaxing being at the beach. I am enjoying just sitting by the ocean day after day, feet in the water, head in the clouds, the womb-like thrash of the ocean waves in my ears.

My uncle and his family came to the beach one day, and
I swam in the water like a giddy eight year old. There have been hard moments this week too.

A person we recently met dropped by, and when I confided to her that I was trying with great difficulty to have children, she told me that maybe God didn't intend me to have children. At that moment, I felt slapped down by her proclamation.

Thankfully, exactly at that moment, an odd thing happened that seemed to save me: three little girls with dark curly hair walked by, looking much the way I envision my future daughter will look.

I grabbed the sight of those little girls as a sign that maybe I am intended to have kids--dare I hope, maybe even a daughter--and I should ignore my neighbor's careless comment. I stayed focused on the girls and slapped her words out of my head.

My young cousin Chuck slept over. One night, Chris and Chuck all went down to the amusement center. Once we got there, we all started acting like kids, running, skipping, acting crazy. In that moment, a snapshot of the three of us running to the center imprints on my memory. I think: if it turns out I am pregnant, this night marks the beginning of something new and different in my life.

The next day, at about 1 in the afternoon, I was hit with a wave of tiredness like a tiredness I have never felt before. I laid down and actually slept for three hours.

Since I never nap, this was quite different for me. My body was so exhausted. Could it be???? I dare not analyze this too much, but I pray and keep up my optimism.

The waiting is hard. When people say that maybe God doesn't want me to have children, I want to scream. 'Why???? Why do you say that? Why do you think that God would not want me to have children?'

Why is it so easy to automatically think God is all about denying and withholding, when the Bible speaks mostly about God's great love and how if we have faith, we can move mountains?

It is a disgrace that people are so quick to think of God as a chiding schoolmaster, who would rather rap you on the knuckles and deny any and all requests, rather than being the loving kind merciful God He is.

This whole process of trying to get pregnant sometimes reminds me of a time when I was younger, and deeply in love with a man who didn't love me back, or who loved me sometimes, and didn't love me other times. Back then, friends would say things like, "I don't think you two were meant to be" and I bucked it.

They ended up being right.

I still sometimes wonder why. Why wasn't that relationship meant to be? How could I love someone so much and him not feel the same way in return? Is having children going to end up being just like that episode in my life--something I desperately want and yearn for, only to have the answer be no?

I feel so alone right now. What will I do if I'm not pregnant? Get sperm from someone other than my husband? Someone whose sperm is more compatible with mine? A guy with stronger sperm? At this point, I just want a child and I'm beginning not to care how I get it. Should I adopt a child? I can hardly bear another month to pass.

For now, I sit by the ocean, and wait. My 96 year old grandmother Maria teases me, and tells me to sit down and let the ocean water float into my vagina. She knows I'm trying to get pregnant (she doesn't know about the infertility treatments--how in the world would I explain them to a 94 year old woman from Italy.)

She says the water will help my body be strong and will help me get pregnant. I do what she says, laughing, but secretly hoping that my wise beautiful grandmother is right, and that the strength of the ocean strengthens my tired body enough to get pregnant.

For The Love of My Mother

I am sitting on the beach late this afternoon, wondering (as usual..so what's new) if I am pregnant or not.

If I think about it, I have to admit that a part of me doesn't think I deserve to have a baby.

In fact, most of the time, I don't feel like I deserve even the smallest of things, never mind the one thing in this world I want most.

I realized, as I was sitting by the ocean, that for me to help my body get pregnant, I need to trick my body into thinking it is doing this for my mother, and not myself.

From now on, in an attempt to trick my body into giving me what I want, I am going to tell my body that it must rise up and produce a baby for my mother. Body, we must do this for my mother.

I need a motivation outside of myself for this to work.

I know my mother would love to be a grandmother. Recently, my mother ran into the mother of one of my childhood friends. This woman, who has three grandchildren, announced to my mother, "Sally, you don't know how wonderful it is to have a grandchild. Just think, you are the only one (out of this group of friends) who isn't a grandmother."

Talk about insensitive. Maybe this lady meant no harm, but I know it hurt my mother to think that most of my childhood friends have babies and I do not.

I have to have children, so this will be the last time some petty, mean-spirited, or just plain clueless person will have ammunition to hurt my mother again.

I will not allow my mother to arrive at her old age without grandchildren.

Never do I want my mother to feel that because of my failures, she ended up missing out on one of life's grand last-minute surprises.

I don't want my mother to pity me, or herself, because we are babyless people.

As I focus my thoughts on my mother, I can actually feel my body getting stronger.

For myself, I probably won't allow my body to be strong enough to make a baby.

For my mother, I can put aside my own self-loathing long enough to let my body do its natural thing and make a baby.

I saw how sad my mother was when this woman alluded to the fact that all my friends from childhood have been successful enough to make a baby, and I, the only freak in the group, still does not have a baby.

Nope, I'm sick of being a freak who causes my mother pain. I have to do something normal her sake.

Why should she look at other women and feel they are rewarded in some way that she is not?

To make this happen, I need to keep focusing on my mother and not myself.

For myself, my body will say: "You are too bad of a person to ever get what you want."

But for my mother, my body will be better than it naturally is.

When I think of my mother, the uneasiness in my stomach disappears and is replaced by something much clearer I can't fully explain.

I feel stronger.

My body wants to do right by my mother. I sit on the beach, inhaling the sun and air, and hope and strength return to the self-hating me.

Because I love my mother so much, I will create a grandchild for her.

I'm tired of being the freaky, quirky, odd daughter she always has to apologize for.

I'm hoping that my body will agree that even if I don't deserve a baby, my mother certainly deserves a grandchild.

Friday Came

Chris left for work early this morning. Since there is no phone here at the beach cottage, I will have to use the pay phone at the convenience store down the street to call my answering machine at home later today to hear the nurse's message. I could go home and wait for the message, but since we have only one car, I would be stuck there all day today and tomorrow, and I don't want to be sitting at home waiting to hear no.

Most of the day, I sat by the ocean. The waves crashing and diving up and down the beach massage the weary part of me. Being here has been more relaxing than I ever imagined.

There have even been moments I almost forget about my desperation to have a baby. Well, not really moments, but maybe a minute or two of peace, here and there. The ocean can do that, give even the saddest most desperate person, a few moments of peace.

Today, I am fidgety all day. The nurse will call by 4 o'clock, as they always do. I wish 4 o'clock would just come and be over with. I know what it coming. I want it done.

Four o'clock comes. I borrow some change from my mother and I walk down the concrete sidewalk to the convenience store. This is the same convenience store where my cousin Sheri and I used to hang out at as budding teenagers. We would stand in the store's parking lot, preening, flirting, enjoying the teenage world of cute boys and shy smiles.

It is the same store where as a 12-year old girl, I stood outside the door and asked customers to sign a petition to bring back the 100-year old merry-go-round that developers sold to an amusement park in San Diego that had graced Salisbury center since the.

I loved that carousel as a child. I can still see myself trying to grab the gold ring. I felt so powerful back then, so naively powerful as to think a silly petition would make the owners of the carousel give up whatever profits they seized from the sale and return the carousel back to its rightly place at the center.

How odd that now I walk to this store feeling anything but powerful-- did my 12 year old self ever imagine that life would return me to this store, on this day, in this way, to do this task, to hear this news, to feel this way?

Thank God we cannot see the future. The spirited little entrepreneur with the petition! What has become of her? A shadow self enters the parking lot, a pathetic desperate woman bearing no trace to the hardy girl with the petition that once came here.

I go to the pay phone and there is someone on it. I wait. Finally it is free.

I put in the coins, and begin to dial the number that will tell me whether I am pregnant or not.

I stop. I cannot do it. I cannot bear to hear the news. Not here, not surrounded by all the memories of this place. I hang up, press the return button, get my change, and head back down the concrete sidewalk to the beach cottage. Better that I don't know. Better that I stay wondering a little longer. Better that I allow a tiny bit of hope in me to stay alive a bit longer, because I might go completely crazy here in this parking lot if the answer is no. One more day of not knowing is okay, a reprieve from all the hard choices facing me.

I walk back to the cottage. I did the right thing. I could not bear to hear that no over the phone, in the old parking lot where I hung out as a teenager, with people coming and going, buying beer, candy, chips.

I will go home tomorrow and listen to the message alone, with no one around to see me fall apart. I don't think my parents, or the store's patrons, could take seeing the rage that is inside me if the answer is no.

A little girl that once had hope in everything used to hang out here, and she didn't deserve to have her heartbroken in a place where she once felt so strong.

Friday Night Longing

It is a beautiful dark starry summer night and I feel anything but carefree.

Tomorrow I will go home to listen to my answering machine and find out the news. Bad news, I am pretty sure. The answer is going to be no. I know it. The answer for me is always no. I have learned that whenever I really want something, ultimately the answer always turns out to be no. I have come to understand that when I really want something, or someone, truly love this person, this thing, this whatever, the answer is no. So I already know the answer to the question I am waiting to hear answered. How else could it be?

I can barely stand to think of my future right now.

It is Friday night and my cousin Susan has come to visit us. Susan is one of my favorite persons on this earth, and yet tonight, even her visit isn't cheering me up. Susan had her children young in the most beautiful and normal way people are suppose to have children. She is surrounded by children, grandchildren, and right now, in her presence, I feel woefully inadequate.

On my father's side of the family, it seems the tree bears fruit, in the normal way the cycle of life is suppose to work. Childbearing, getting pregnant, having children, comes easily, naturally, the family growing and multiplying. No one is alone or freakish. Life blossoms beautifully. They are part of the normal life continuum.

Susan doesn't know I'm going to an infertility clinic. She might vaguely suspect I want children, but she has no idea that tonight I feel like the biggest failure in the world in her presence. She was a grandmother at 36. Here I am, 33 years old and still no children. I once thought waiting until you were older to have children was the thing to do, and now I realize that the tables have turned and actually I am the unnatural freak who missed the biological boat.

Susan, my parents and myself go down to the center to get some fried dough and pizza.

The "center" as we call this part of the beach is to an outsider nothing but a honky tonk bunch of neon signs, fried food, men in tattoos wearing leather jackets and girls with store bought bleached hair and too little clothes. But to my family, the center is a place of beautiful, never-to-be forgotten memories, of amusement park rides and favorite ice creams, the bright lights thrilling us in the darkness. It is the place where me and my cousins Sheri and Tina roamed around as teenagers, enjoying the tiny element of danger the night held, along with the ice cream and moon pies at Willy's, and most of all, the camaraderie of family.

Usually, staying at my favorite beach in the world, one laden with such glorious childhood memories, and having my beloved cousin Susan sleep over, would feel like a great and grand treat.

But tonight, the world feels ugly and sad to me. I am too old to be longing for the past. I should be over wanting and yearning for what used to be by now. Everywhere I look tonight, the past feels so much better than the present or even the future. It seems that at 12 years old, I had more than I have now--more connection, more family, more love, more fun. A child would bring it all back, change the life I have now. In the presence of my cousin who had four children by the time she was my age, I feel dull, barren, like a wrinkled fruit that never fully ripened. I live my life missing the past, and I'm tired of that...Tired of looking back all the time. I want a reason, a someone, to look forward for. I need someone to create new memories for, rather than yearning for people and memories long gone in my life.

I want a child to introduce me to a new way of being, and reconnect with an old way of being that I have lost.

I want to be part of the club. That's it...I want to be a member in the natural process of life. I want to do what people, animals, bugs, birds, and all living beings have been doing since the earth came into existence.

Trees have leaves, squirrels have baby squirrels, from dirt comes weeds, plants and flowers, the sky gives out rain and ants breed more ants, and even old trees find a way to resurrect themselves in the spring to heave out a few more twigs and a few more leaves. Then, why is having a baby so hard for me?

Why, from the beginning, has everything about creating my own family been hard for me, from getting married to now having a baby? Why is this natural part of life such a struggle for me? My cousins seem to get married and have children without barely a thought, they so fit in the natural cycle of life, and yet for me, having my own family is a grueling, frustrating, nearly impossible dream.

I sat in the car while my parents and Susan went to get pizza at a place we've been going for years. I feel too sad to enjoy pizza or even get my body to move out of the car.

I stay in the car while they get in line for the pizza--I cannot bring myself to participate in the buzz of life going on around me tonight, when there is no buzz in my life that even remotely mirrors what is happening in the center tonight or what has happened here for generations.

I cannot help but thinking that by the time Susan was my age, she had given birth four times. I remember her at my age--she was all mother, all grown-up, a part of life's process. She had a family, a definite somewhere to belong in this world.

I sit in the car, watching all the life around me, the life I used to believe I would have long ago when I came here as a child. I feel like such a failure right now. The drizzle starts to fall and my heart is slowly and dully breaking.

News Arrives

Today I woke up with one thought in my mind: get out of here before you get the news. I'm am a raging volcano ready to explode.

If I call my house, check my answering machine, and hear' no, sorry-you-are-not-pregnant, I am going to flip out'. No, I am going to die. I am going to blame everyone around me for my life, for my lonely existence in a childless world. So this morning, I made some excuse about needing to go home to do some work on my online magazine, and I borrowed my mother's red Toyota Camry.

The drive home was fast, as I live only about 35 minutes from the beach. The Toyota ran so smoothly I felt like I was flying. I drive a clunky old Volvo, and I'm not used to this feeling of gliding down the highway. The ride home, so mockingly free, gave me a reprieve from my pain.

When I got home, I went straight up to our office where the answering machine lives. The red button was not blinking. I pressed play. Nothing. No message.

What happened is clear: my husband came home, played out the sad message of no, and decided not to save it, so as to spare me the pain. He wants to tell me himself.

He is right. I feel better not hearing it. I like the silence. I've heard enough no's loud and clear in my life. I don't want to hear no again. My husband is kind, and I feel a dull sense of relief, although I know this means terrible choices wait ahead for me.

We've done seven IUIs now, and I'm growing more convinced that the reason I can't get pregnant is that my eggs and my husband's sperm don't want to mate. What next? Look for somebody else's sperm? A pretty immoral idea, but not one I haven't toyed with.

My husband says fine, go do what you want, and a part of me screams yes, I deserve to be able to find a better biological choice, because above all else, I want children. Terrible. Horrible thoughts. I would never actually do something so immoral, but this is where sadness can lead: to desperate ideas that are wrong and that I would never do.

I get on my computer, one of the few places in this world where serenity comes over me.

I am working on my online magazine, and I have met an amazing web designer named Ann Sowers who is going to redesign the site.

When I'm working on Commitment, I become enraptured, in flow, and my thoughts of bearing children are replaced with creative thrill for a short time.

When I work on my magazine, I escape, if just for a few minutes, from being the washed out failure I am. I am dashing out West in my covered wagon, towards a new life.

Working on Commitment always calms me down. A few hours pass and it is almost time to get back to the beach.

I'm going to hear no tonight. Right out loud tonight I will hear no.

But at least it will be from my husband, and not from the voice of a nurse doing her routine calls, who says 'no, you are not pregnant' with the same kind of faux sympathy of a salesgirl who tells you, no, that blouse is no longer on sale, but try back next week.

I need to get back to the beach.

The Answer Comes

I am sitting in the kitchen at the beach cottage. Early evening has come and a light darkness sprinkles the world. We have plans tonight with our friends Melanie and Darren. I am waiting for everyone to arrive. It is getting dark and my husband walks in.

"Did you hear the news?" he says casually.

"No," I answered, immediately starting to hate him. It is easy to blame him, hate him, consider it all is his fault that I have to endure this.

"You are pregnant," he says, almost matter-of-factly.

I stop. "You are lying," I blurt out.

"I'm not," he says. "I thought you knew. The nurse called. She said you are pregnant."

I am stunned. Happy. Disbelieving. Shocked. Not sure I'm ready to believe it.

"Then why didn't you save the message for me?" I retort, challenging this notion.

"Because I thought you heard it Friday night. So when I got home I didn't save it. I thought you knew," he explained.

I sat stunned for a few moments, still not fully comprehending this. Then the world changes hue and a different color comes over everything. The universe has shifted, in the way I had begged and pleaded and waited for. A new and different door has opened for me and something that resembles calm, gratitude, and quiet jubiliance enters my soul.

Yes, there was optimism this cycle. Momentum was definitely building. I even felt joy during certain moments. Hadn't I prayed constantly? I know God hears prayers and maybe He heard my prayer.

Still I couldn't let myself believe that yes had finally arrived.

My husband then told me the nurse said I had to go for three more pregnancy tests to be sure.

Always more tests...Three more tests.

Only in the world of infertility does 'yes you are pregnant' also mean you need three more tests to ABSOLUTELY BE SURE you are pregnant.

I am shocked and happy. Maybe I was even expecting this. I had begged God so much, perhaps He heard me. Perhaps he saw me last month throwing myself on the side of the road crying, and He wanted to help me.

Melanie and Darren arrive. We sort of blurt out the news to everyone-- my parents, Melanie, my grandmother. Everyone is happy, but they seem dazed and shocked too.

You would imagine this would be a big night of celebration. I suppose now you expect a few pages about the glorious night I enjoyed with family and friends, celebrating the fact that I was finally pregnant.

But instead fear rose up in me. Fear rose up in my husband. After months and months of stress, we were not accustomed to hearing yes.

We were so accustom to disappointment and anger, it didn't feel quite natural yet to sit back and enjoy.

We all went out to dinner, and the problem started with a bowl of soup.

At first, I ordered a bowl of soup, but then I saw the steak, and decided to get that instead. We were on a tight budget and so I asked the waitress to cancel the soup. Well, the order came, and she brought the steak and the soup. I told her I didn't want the soup, and she said it was too late to send it back.

If I had the money, I would have simply paid for the soup--but I didn't have the money for both, (going to acupuncture so many times depleted our budget) and I proceeded to get into an argument with her over the bill. No, I told her, I am not paying for the soup. She was snappy back at me. We went back and forth, until finally she took the soup off the bill, but not before saying something nasty about me.

Now, instead of backing me, my husband got really angry at me. He was (boo hoo) embarrassed.

I wanted to say, is it not my fault we don't have the money for both. And so a big fight between us began. He thought I was rude and immature. I thought he was a wimp for not standing up for me. How could he not defend me, when I was carrying his child? On the way home, all our pent-up rage and exhaustion from the past few weeks exploded into a rip-roaring fight. He wished he wasn't having a baby with me! I wished I wasn't having a baby with him!

All the fight in us burst open and tumbled out and we said some horrible things. I think the fact that we had been walking on pins and needles around this IUI for so long wore us out.

We got back to the beach cottage and went to bed.

Looking back, I don't think I felt comfortable allowing myself to feel the joy that was rightfully mine that night.

I expected to hear no and had gotten so used to hearing no, that a very destructive part of me needed to make trouble because pain and trouble was what I was accustomed to.

You would think that now that I finally had what I wanted for so long I would be happy, but that is the beauty of being a human--the paradoxical feelings that can exist within one person. Just a month ago, I was throwing myself on the side of a road, crying with agony, because no baby had arrived for me yet. Now, a month later, I am pregnant and I'm scared of having a baby with my husband, and I'm not sure I'm ready. I want it, the baby, so much, and yet I am scared.

This whole infertility process up to this point made us both a bit insane--the whole trying/not getting/trying/not getting/ and now finally, when we didn't expect it, getting. We had both been so hurt and so disappointed for so long, and now a yes. Did we deserve this yes? Were we ready for this change?

But when I woke up the next day, everything was already feeling very different.

Yes, Its True

I am pregnant. Let me say again those three long-awaited magic words: I am pregnant.

Yahoo! Yipee! Who cares about last night's fight? Who cares about anything? I, me, the person I am, is actually and really pregnant.

I need to go for three more tests, but that doesn't matter. I am truly pregnant. Thank you God. I am going to be a Mom!

The world looks like a different place today. The sun shines differently, the breeze blows differently, I look in the mirror and see myself differently...I am pregnant! I am pregnant! I am pregnant!

I Am A Pregnant Lady

I still can't believe I am pregnant!

It is a week after we got the good news. I am walking around dazed and happy.

I have to get two more tests to confirm that officially I am pregnant, but once I have those tests, I am officially on the way to having my baby!

I never felt more important and more wonderfully ordinary in my entire life.

I am finally part of humanity's drumbeat, a note heard in the universal rhythm of life, life going on, life beating heart.

Let me shout it from the roof top--I AM PREGNANT!

We returned home from the beach after we got the good news. My parents are still there on vacation and we went for a visit today. When we get there, my mother's best friend Lydia was visiting. It felt so exciting to share the news with her.

I could tell my parents felt so proud too...so proud to be part of something so normal.

My mother already bought me a baby name book. I immediately start flipping through it admiring all the beautiful baby names.

I feel like I'm finally part of life's parade, one of the marchers, no longer forced to sit on the sidelines cheering for all the others passing me by with a march of their own. I am going to have a place in this world, a starring role, and that will be of a mother.

A Third Yes!

Today was the third test to determine if I am pregnant. The day started out beautiful and sunny, and I had a good feeling.

I drove to the clinic about 6 a.m. It felt good to be there, and in a strange way, I've come to really enjoy this place and the people.

Carol did my blood test and was excited for me. As I was walking out to the elevator, I thought that if I am pregnant, I will miss this place.

Then I came home, did some chores, and decided to watch, "All My Children" before I had to leave for work—something I almost never do.

Oddly enough a character on the show, Liza, found out she was pregnant today. I started to cry, and felt that maybe this was a good sign, if not a very odd coincidence.

If I am pregnant, I will always remember that Liza found out she was pregnant the same day I did.

I left for work, and knew that by the time I got to work around 4 o'clock, the answer would be waiting on my answering machine.

I got into work, went to my desk, dialed my home number to check my messages, and yes, the nurse said, all my numbers were right: I am pregnant. Three tests and all confirm: I am most definitely and completely pregnant.

A loud hooray is going off in my brain. Louder than probably any hooray I've ever experienced in my life before.

I'm not sure quite why the first test was not enough, but in the world of infertility...everything is slightly different.

I immediately logged off my computer, went into the conference area, and wrote my baby a letter, with the exact time and date on it.
Then I called Chris at work. I could hear all his friends at the salon congratulating him.

My friend Bonnie overheard me and gave me a big congratulations hug in the bathroom. Then I told my boss George, and asked if they had shields to protect me from radioactive waves from the computer. He said no, so I'll try to find out to buy to protect me.

What a great day!

But tonight, as usual after hearing good news, Chris and I fought.

We should have been so close tonight, but instead, after a long day at work, we sat at the kitchen table and bickered over this and that.

Strange, because we tried so hard to get pregnant and now we are fighting and stressed because we got what we worked so hard for. We are happy and angry, excited and scared out of our minds. The infertility treatments have made us tired and in some ways, we see one another as the enemy now. I blamed his sperm. He blamed me for being so driven to have a baby that I ignored our relationship.

I don't care, however--because bottom line is I want a baby more than I want anything else in this world and I'm actually pregnant!!!! He is not the issue right now. Little by little, the agitation left, the fight ended, and I went to bed thanking God.

Being Pregnant

The first few months of my pregnancy have been about being cautious. I am on a bed rest to ensure a healthy delivery, meaning I have to take it easy. I have taken a leave from work.

The first obstetrician I had was a difficult personality for me, but it wasn't until my best friend Cindy told me, "if you leave someone's presence feeling afraid, that is a signal to get away from that person."

So I listened, followed my gut instinct, and somehow found the exactly right doctor for my personality. He agreed to do all the tests I needed, and immediately gave me the documentation I needed to continue on bed rest.

He even scheduled weekly ultrasounds at the hospital to monitor my baby's progress. No more wondering if my baby is okay!

Wow, I am relieved. This is the kind of doctor I have needed for a long time. I'm glad Cindy forced me to listen to my feelings about my ob/gyn--if you walk away feeling bad about an experience, that is usually a sign that something is wrong and the warning should be heeded. Thank you Cindy!

It's A Girl!

My doctor wants to ease my worries over my baby, so he scheduled a high resolution ultrasound this morning at a local hospital. A technician from the Boston area came to do it.

It was thrilling, a relief, and totally mind-boggling all at once to learn that my baby's heart had formed correctly, that the spine was formed and aligned properly, that the kidneys looked good, and that it appears that there is no sign of down syndrome. Not that it would matter, but it was a relief to learn that as far as the technician could see, my baby was healthy.

My baby is healthy! I say a quick prayer of thanks to God.

Then the technician asked me, "Do you want to know the sex?"

I hesitated, and asked my husband if he thought we should find out. "It is up to you," he said kindly.

"Yes," I whispered. I was convinced I was having a boy. I don't know why, but I assumed my baby was a boy. Maybe because, in my heart, I desperately want my first child to be a girl, so I assume that whenever I desperately want something, I'll get something else.

I also am reminded of what my husband said, that God would probably never give me a girl, and even though that nasty fight is behind us, his words stay with me. On some level, I too believe that I probably don't deserve a girl...

"It's a girl!" the technician blurted out.

"Are you sure?" I asked, not daring to believe it.

"I am absolutely sure," she said.

Oh my God, a girl! A girl! A girl! A girl! A girl! A GIRL! A GIRL! I want to shout it from the rooftops! Have it announced on the evening news! Ring every bell in every city!

A daughter...can you imagine me, me-- actually having a daughter? My daughter...has there ever been two more beautiful words in the English language or any language?Have two words in the history of humankind ever been more significant? More beautiful? More life-changing? More profound? I am in a daze. A cozy, warm haze forms around me. I am in a cocoon, as I began the transformation into a new life as mother of a daughter! MY DAUGHTER! Me? Can I really have this? A confirmation from God that He doesn't hate me. A divine high-five that He allowed me to actually conceive a daughter. My husband was wrong...God wasn't going to punish me by never giving me the daughter of my dreams...I am actually receiving what I wanted the most.

A son would be amazing someday, but first, I need a girl, a daughter, to share my life journey with.

Someday I will be ready and anxious for a son. But for now, all I have ever wanted was a daughter.

A daughter...a daughter! my daughter...my daughter...I can't say the words enough. I feel a ticklish thrill! I keep a journal about my pregnancy and tonight I started my entry with, "To my daughter:"

My daughter....two words more profound than all the works of Shakespeare.

My baby...my daughter...my daughter is healthy! MY DAUGHTER! HOORAY! THANK YOU GOD! Her heart is strong! Her spine is okay! Her head is the right size! I am basking in the glow of this new life that I am walking towards and who is coming towards me.
God is not denying me what I have wanted more than anything else in this world. Maybe I am not such a rotten person after all. Maybe I will actually get what I want for once.

My daughter...no words have ever been spoken on this planet that could be more beautiful to me.

My Routine

There is a comfortable and joyful quietness to the rhythm of my life right now. I go few places. I mostly stay home, work on my online magazine, welcome occasional visits from friends and watch TV.

I haven't felt this protected since I was a child. I've never had a time in my adulthood where so little was expected of me and where I am the recipient of so much love and goodwill. My husband massages my feet every night. Chelsea mails me homemade cards and gifts to cheer me up. Roz, who is overseas in Armenia waiting to adopt her little girl, wrote and said she is praying for me. This is a happy, happy time for me. I still worry at times. I am very, very careful. I don't eat anything that could possibly harm my baby. I juice spinach every day, and when I don't feel like drinking it, I say to myself, "good for my baby girl...good for my baby girl...good for my baby girl" and it goes right down.

My husband and I, after living here a few years, have a group of friends who come over our house a lot. I usually retire to bed early, but my husband stays up playing cards with Lenny and Matthew. We have wonderful neighbors, like Richard, Janice and Helene, who are the perfect neighbors for me.

Infertility was so hard and long. Having this baby is the culmination of so many dreams. Now I wait, and try to enjoy the wait. It is a blissful, peaceful, quiet time.

Fourth Month

 I have reached the four month mark of my pregnancy. Now that I've successfully reached the three month mark, I am feeling more comfortable.
Knowing I am having a girl, and seeing the high resolution ultrasound and learning that somehow, miraculously, she has a heart and a spine that has formed correctly, is giving me comfort. I am also feeling a lot less anxious, since I have a doctor I like and he is checking on the baby with weekly ultrasounds

Life has taken on a different, warmer, rosier glow.

Now that we are at the four month mark, my daughter's ears have grown enough that she has developed the ability to hear. So I tape recorded a message to her that I play every night. I put the earphones on my stomach, and play 30 minutes of Mozart to her, and then I change the tape and play my message to her.

When I play the tape to her, an amazing sense of contentment, unlike anything I've ever experienced before, envelopes me. In my message, I tell her about all the wonderful things we are going to do together...Honey, we are going to bake cookies together. We are going to spend lots of time at the beach jumping waves and building sand castles. We are going to build a tree house, read wonderful children's stories, have sunny Friday afternoon picnics, and fall completely in love with each other.

Corny, I know. Sappy as anything. Over-the-top sentimental. God, I love her so much.

Then I play her the message my husband taped to her, where he talks about how much he loves her and is excited to see her.

Usually I fall asleep by 8 p.m.

This routine appears so mundane, but for me it is pure excitement--a new door opening that had been closed for such a long time.
It is not only the beginning of my daughter's life, but also the start of my life as a mother.

I still feel afraid at times. There are still moments when I worry a lot.

I am very careful. I don't eat restaurant-cooked meats.
I stay away from cheese. I juice spinach every day, and I take chlorophyll because I read somewhere that it is healthy for pregnant women. I take three folic acid vitamins a day, plus a prenatal vitamin. And I pray, and I pray. I pray constantly that my baby lives and grows.

A daughter is coming to me. Praise God. Somehow the heavens have opened to me. How did this happen?

How did I actually get pregnant and conceive a daughter who has a heart that is working properly, and a head and a spine that formed exactly as they should? How did I get to this place, where I sleep and relax in a bedroom with the prettiest green color walls on earth, with my baby growing inside me listening to my voice, her father's voice and Mozart's majestic music, every night?

Getting pregnant was so hard for me. Wrenching. A continuation of many years of disappointments, but the bitterest denial of all. So I take nothing for granted. Not a day do I complain. I have never felt happier, more content, than I do now.

Ever since I was pregnant, it seems the world around me has opened their arms with support and comfort from all directions.

A year ago, this life would not have seemed possible. How did this happen to me? Could it be true?

After a long bloody nightmare, I am living a dream. At night, when I'm playing this tape, I feel like I am beginning a new chapter in my life that is the start of a happy-ever-after fairy tale, not a blighted tragedy.

Gray Day in Pregnancy

It is a gray day in every sort of way. My pregnancy these past few months has been wonderful. My new doctor, Dr. Michel Lirrette, is the best doctor in absolutely every way.

Because he knows of my nervousness, he ordered weekly ultrasounds at a nearby hospital for me. It is a routine I have come to love.
I leave the house by 7:30 a.m. and drive about seven minutes to the hospital on the hill where I will deliver my baby. I park not far from the door, enter the cheerful hospital lobby, and go up to the third floor. Ah-- the maternity floor. I love when the elevator doors swing open and I enter the maternity zone. Babies! Babies in the nursery window!

 I can hardly believe that my baby will someday be in that nursery. The nurses are always so nice. I am brought into a room and lie down on a comfortable bed where I am hooked up to monitors that chart my baby's heart. The nurses are always so reassuring.

Yes, she is doing great. Yes, look how strong her heart is. Yes, yes, yes-- your baby is okay. I leave each Wednesday morning feeling relief and joy. And for a little while, all my fears and insecurities disappear. Every week, things get easier. Until today.

Usually, my baby girl is quite active. She kicks a lot, and I do what the nurse recommended in always trying to make sure I feel ten kicks a day. Normally, that is pretty easy.

But today, she is still. So very still. Eerily still. I keep hoping and thinking that at any minute she will start kicking like she always does, but there is nothing--no kicks, no movement at all.

I cannot shake the feeling that something is wrong.

I tell myself that by lunch she will kick. By 2 p.m. she will kick. By 3 p.m. Still nothing. No movement at all. I am getting scared. It is 5 o'clock and she still hasn't kicked all day. I can't get the idea out of my head that maybe something is wrong. Why isn't she moving?

I am far enough along in my pregnancy that if something is wrong, they could take her out and she would survive. Oh God, is she dying inside of me? I've heard too many horror stories to take anything for granted.

Ever since I got pregnant, there have been so many times, like today, that I wish I had given birth when I was a naive 18 year old who knew little about the whole birth-and-babies process.

At that age, you don't know enough to be scared, and you are young enough that most of the time, not a whole lot goes wrong. I think of one of my neighbors who was 18 and didn't know she was pregnant until almost four months into her pregnancy. Four months of no ultrasounds, no folic acid vitamins, no juicing spinach, and with just 30 minutes of labor, she delivered a beautiful, healthy strong baby boy. At one time, I felt bad for girls who had their babies young. Not so much anymore.

As the day wore on, the sky is looking grayer and grayer, I am getting more and more nervous. Is my daughter hanging on for dear life? Is the umbilical cord wound around her neck? My imagination has begun to take me places I don't want to go.

I decide to ask my next door neighbors Richard and Janice for a ride to the hospital, since we only have one car and Chris has taken it to work. I need to have my baby checked, just in case. By now I've learned that better safe than sorry. Sure, they say. I can tell they think I am being paranoid, but still they are ready to help. Please God, please God, please. I pray fervently. At moments like this, I realize that all the tests in the world and all the best doctors in the world cannot compare to believing God is there to listen. Please God, I pray, please save my baby.

113

Please save my baby...these words have echoed in my heart and soul and traveled right up to heaven perhaps ten thousand times since I became pregnant. And now today again, these same words pour out of me.

Right as Richard and Janice come out to drive me to the hospital, my husband pulls in the driveway. Thank you God.

"What is going on?" he asks concerned.

I tell him how I haven't felt the baby move all day, and how the hospital is waiting for us to come. He doesn't hesitate for a minute. "Let's go," he says seriously.

It is moments like this that I am so grateful for my husband. Another man, perhaps a more logical, man, would put aside my fears and worries and convince me not to run off to the hospital.

But my husband didn't blink. If his unborn child has not moved all day, to the hospital we go without a moment's hesitation.

At the hospital, I am immediately hooked up to the fetal monitor. What if my baby has died? I let myself think that for a moment and a feeling so completely dreadful washes over me I have to stop.

I pray and pray, and if not for the comfort of prayer, I might completely loose my mind, especially as the ultrasound begins and the nurse says nothing. Why is the nurse saying nothing?

"What is happening?" I ask the nurse.

"I can't tell yet," she says.

I begin to cry, "Tell me please, is my daughter okay? Did you get a heartbeat?"

I am impatient, demanding, ready to scream.

Finally, after a long minute of silence that seemed like a century, the nurse says, "Your baby is fine."

"We wish all babies that come in here have hearts that beat so strong," she says.

"Is her heart really strong?" I ask, beaming, relieved that yes, my daughter's heart is beating strong.

"Very strong. We would wish that all babies were that healthy," she repeats.

Thank you God! Thank you God. Thank you God. My husband and I leave the hospital beaming, relieved, and happy.

This short scare made me vow to be all the more vigiliant in getting the rest I need and eating healthy. .

Thank God I have a doctor like Dr. Lirrette, who immediately upon receiving my phone call told me to go to the hospital to be checked. Thank God for my neighbors Richard and Janice who were so willing to drive me to the hospital.

Thank God for my husband, who didn't make me feel like an idiot for wanting to have my baby checked. Thank God for the nurse who reassured me so completely by saying my daughter's heart was strong.

To imagine how this night might have gone, it is too much. I know there are women who have faced the unimaginable.

I crawl into bed tonight, exhausted but happy. The gray day is over.

Beautiful April 10 Baby Shower

The months before my baby's birth now seem shrouded by a warm fuzzy sunshine glow. The quiet joys of this pregnancy and the intense love I have received from those around me culminated into a baby shower that turned out to be one of the best days of my life.

On April 10, my mother threw me the most perfect and beautiful baby shower in the clubhouse at my grandmother's apartment complex. My grandmother Maria and I are very close, and having this shower at her place meant a lot to me.

It turned out to be one of the most perfect days of my life--so perfect, it was like I wrote a script detailing what a perfect day in my life would be like. Lots of balloons, a big pink cake, relatives and friends from the various parts of my life and of course, presents.

Lots and lots of wonderful presents: little pink dresses, a child size wicker rocking chair, a jumper with cherries on it, hand-crochet afghans. I wore a beautiful yellow dress with flowers, thanks to a gift certificate given to Chris and I by our friend Matthew. This dress was so joyful and beautiful, it seemed to embody the day we experienced.

The day started early that morning with my next door neighbor Helene bringing me flowers, and ended that night, with me lying in bed, with all the beautiful little dresses and outfits given to me at the shower hanging in my closet.

Leah arrived at my house with candies for me. My cousin Susan gave me a beautiful little white wicker rocking chair, and balloons. Her daughters, my cousins Sheri, Dina, Johnna and Bethany, gave me a beautiful white bassinet. Judy sent an afghan made by her mother.

My mother prepared stuffed shells and bought a huge beautiful cake with pink and white icing. So many friends and family were there...Aunt Betty, cousin Denise, Aunt Angie, Aunt Sandra, Aunt Rose, Leslie, Elaine, Judy, Leslie, on and on it went. My mother went all out with this shower and did so much work to make it spectacular for me. She made so much food. I love my Mom so much.

I looked so big that at the shower, my Aunt Angie thought I might be giving birth soon.

Sitting at the table with Chris, my mother, Aunt Betty and Aunt Angie, was a feeling of closeness I have not felt in such a long time.

The sun shined in the most spectacular spring way all day.

My little girl was coming soon!

That night, Chris went out with our friends Melanie and Darren, Tyrone and Lenny, and I stayed home. Every few minutes, I would jump up from my bed, run to my closet and look at all the pretty clothes that were given to my daughter that day.

I did this for hours.

Every few minutes, I would get up from bed and run to the closet to look at all the cute little dresses and adorable outfits. I kept pinching myself figuratively--my little girl would soon wear those dresses! Then, I'd get out of bed again, run over to the closet, touch the dresses and all the outfits, and feel almost giddy with glee.
I knew from that night on that never again would my life be as lonely as it had been before. A little girl--my little girl—was going to wear those dresses! She is almost here!

A new life was beginning for me...Then out of the bed I'd pop again, run over to the closet to touch and look one more time.

I went to bed with prayers of thanks on my lips and a feeling that this beautiful day was one I will never forget.

My Baby Is Born

On May 17, 1999, the most miraculous thing ever to happen in my life actually occurred: my 8 pound, 11 ounce little girl was born.

"Beautiful like Mommy," Dr. Lirrette declared at 7:30 a.m. on that glorious Monday morning when he pulled her from my stomach and for the first time ever, I laid my eyes upon the loveliest little creature imaginable to have ever come to earth.

It happened. I gave birth to a baby. Me! She made it through the pregnancy!

Yes, I actually conceived and gave birth to a baby. Me! Yes-- actually me. To describe it as wonderful would be a terrible understatement.

The night before, my grandmother Maria prepared a beautiful meal for me, my husband, parents and cousin Susan.

Then, at 5 o'clock the next morning, we went to the hospital.

My Dad, Mom and cousin Susan were all there, waiting for us. They had come to be there for my daughter's birth.

While I was getting my epidural, a very wonderful nurse named Mary held me and asked, 'do you want to say a prayer?' I nodded. Her kindness got me through a rough moment.

Then, I laid there waiting to feel some pain.

Friends had told me to expect a lot of tugging during the caesarean, so I waited for the tug.

Suddenly, there was Dr. Lirrette, swinging around saying, "she's beautiful like Mommy" and my daughter had arrived without barely a blink of pain.

She was covered in blood and oh so beautiful. They took her to be cleaned up and I was sent back to my room.

While I waited, my parents, grandmother, and aunts came in. My father was beaming, "she looks so strong," he said.

Then, the most amazing thing happened. When they brought her to me for the first time, I held her and suddenly she held my finger. I could feel a connection between us, sort of like, 'Hi Mom! I know you." She actually was holding my finger! She was connecting to me!

The rest of the day, I was on such a high that despite all the pain medicine I was on, I didn't stop talking, I talked and talked to whomever would listen. I was so happy that all I wanted to do was talk!

My daughter is here! She made it!

My life has never felt sweeter or more complete.

Part II: Secondary Infertility

Having a baby was everything I dreamed it would be and more. To say that my daughter changed my life and gave me a sense of happiness, purpose and belonging that I have always longed for would be an understatement.

All the pain, frustration and difficulty I endured to have her was absolutely and completely worth it. And looking back, it all now seems like a rather beautiful memory because it culminated into the birth of my daughter.

Now I begin another chapter in my book, and it is about the pain and frustration of secondary infertility.

I will acknowledge right now that I am very lucky to have one biological child. I know many people would be overjoyed and content with that. On many levels, I was too. If I had only her, my life would be complete.

Yet, once I had her, I was fueled with an intense and driving desire to have more children. Why? Well, ever since I was young, when I pictured my family, it always included more than one child. I was an only child, and as happy as my childhood was, I wanted to create a different family structure than the exact same one I had. Perhaps I felt that way because I never had siblings, and what we don't have as children, we always want to give our children. Whatever the reason, I desperately wanted my daughter to have a brother or sister.

I also wanted the chance to love more than one child. I wanted four, five, six or more people living in my home. I have always craved hustle, bustle, and noise in my home.

I naively thought that because I had finally conceived and given birth to my daughter that I would easily get pregnant a second time.

A friend recently asked me, 'are you going to try to get pregnant again?' ' 'Yes,' I answered. 'How long do you think it will take?' she asked. And very cavalierly I said, "maybe three or four months." How wrong I was.

This is the irony of secondary infertility. Just because you had a baby the first time, doesn't mean it is going to happen easily the next time.

When my daughter neared a year and a half, my husband and I decided it was time to begin trying for a second child. I saw how outgoing she was, how much she loved other children, and how sometimes she was lonely and needed companionship.

Every week, when I went to story time at a local library with my mother. I saw up close how the children with brothers and sisters enjoyed a sense of security and belonging that my daughter lacked. They didn't seem as desperate or as lonely as she was. They weren't trying to become part of other people's parade, because they had children in their world who belonged to them. Each week, a mother and her three daughters all about a year apart came to story time. I saw how happy they were and how they didn't want for anything or anyone, and I ached for my daughter to have that serene sense of belonging and permanence of a sibling in her life.

Whenever we went to the park, my daughter would get so excited seeing the other children. Sometimes the children were friendly and eager playmates, and sometimes they weren't. That burned. I couldn't stand to see her at the mercy of these kids.

I wanted my daughter to have loving relationships, with a foundation based on family, not on the fickle ups and downs of childhood friendships.

Thus began my uphill battle to give my daughter a sibling, and myself a second child to love.

Secondary infertility can seem trivial, especially to a person going through infertility treatments for the first time. I understand that completely.

Before I had my daughter, I would have scoffed at anyone who pitied themselves for being unable to have a second baby. When you have no child, there is little room for pitying anyone who has one child.

But once I had a child, I felt compelled to create a family structure that included the sibling relationship. I need to add a side note on this: I was an only child, and truthfully, I probably had one of the best and happiest childhoods a kid could wish for.

So if you have one child, don't for a moment be misled into thinking only children are unhappy children—I was an only child and I wouldn't trade my childhood memories and life with anyone, including those with siblings.

The next part of my book will talk about the challenges of secondary infertility. Not being able to have a second child puts you into a certain family structure, and if that family structure is not one you chose, it can be hard to accept.

Secondary infertility is more heart wrenching than imagined. There is less validation for the pain involved. If people tell you God doesn't want you to have a baby the first time, they can't wait to tell you that maybe you were meant to have only one child the second time. Some people, think were already given enough with one baby--who are you to push it and think you deserve two babies. Friends who also suffered with infertility the first time, and are understandably content with their one baby, aren't always keen to give you the encouragement needed to try again.

Here is my experience with secondary infertility. I hope it can help you in some way. My experiences reflect what many of you have gone through, whether you are trying for your first or second baby. I hope it can help or comfort you in some way.

Baby Making With Husband Nowhere In Sight

Today was my third IUI trying for a second child. Today was different than any of the other IUIs I've done before. My husband and I were not even together during the IUI. We went to the clinic at different times, in separate cars.

Because he had to work all day, and there was an ice cream festival at my work that my mother and I were bringing my daughter to, my husband drove to the clinic at 7 a.m., gave his sperm, and went off to work. An hour later, I arrived for my IUI.

How odd, I thought as I was driving to the clinic, I am now going to make a baby with my mother and my daughter, with my husband nowhere in sight. I felt sorry for myself, because as a young teenage girl, I would have never imagined that my baby making experience would include my mother, a nurse, and a speculum that really, really hurt.

Not that the other IUIs have ever felt natural to me, but having my husband at the clinic with me felt at least more normal--at least, I reasoned, we were doing this together.

Imagine how far science had come--that two people can make a baby separated by a few hours and several miles.

Nothing at all romantic about this baby-making exchange.

When I was young, and imagined having children, I never could have imagined that this would my future. Thank God I didn't know it would turn out this way. Thank God no one at 17 ever showed me a crystal ball into my baby-making future. My heart would have been broken. But I want another baby so much, that most of the time I dismiss these sentimental yearnings, I can't let anything interfere with my fertility treatments.

But today the yearnings got me good, and I feel a heavy load of melancholy.

I am so far away from the original way people usually create a family.

Once the IUI was over, my Mom and I drove to the ice cream festival at my workplace, a PBS station in Boston. Some of my co-workers got to meet my daughter for the first time.

As we drove home, my mother turned to me said, "Maybe you are pregnant."

Her hopefulness was sweet.

It must have been weird for my mother to go with me to the clinic, while I went into a room to be impregnated with my husband's sperm.

I can only imagine what my mother was thinking. But my Mom, always brave and tactful, didn't say anything mean or negative.

That night, I told my husband how sad I was that we were not together for today's IUI. He said he felt the same way.

He doesn't take things as passionately as I do, or get as worked up when things don't work out. I think because I had such high expectations for love and romance, that times like this put a spotlight on how far I've travelled from the original dream for my life.

I have to let it go. I know I am so lucky to have my first baby. I could feel it today when I walked into that waiting room with my beautiful daughter and I saw the expressions on the faces of some of the women, and even men, when my daughter and I began to play with some toys. Their eyes lit up--a baby! Their eyes looked sad--a baby!...Someone else's as usual. I remember how I used to feel when someone would come into the waiting room with a baby. I felt excited, resentful, frustrated all at the same time. Sometimes seeing their success in having a baby made me hopeful. Sometimes their success made me jealous. Sometimes I felt all goopy to see a baby and to dare to imagine what it must feel like to have little hands to hold and cheeks to kiss.

I saw in the faces of the couples in the waiting room that same longing, mixed with hopefulness. So I know I shouldn't complain.

Tonight, I want to just snuggle up with my husband, and imagine that I am 17 and still allowed to believe that babies are made in bed by two people madly in love.

Third Try and You're Out?

This month marked my third IUI try, and the answer has been, every single month, has been no.

No.

No.

No.

I'm tired of hearing no.

I thought after my daughter was born that trying for a second baby would be easy, quick and fast.

I thought once I decided it was time for another baby, it would be simple: an IUI, some medication, acupuncture every week, and kazam--a baby!

Now I'm getting nervous. Three IUI tries and no baby? What if I never get pregnant again? It has been three years since my daughter was conceived and two years since she was born.

Every year that goes by means my eggs are older. Maybe I should have tried for another baby when she was six months old. But I was so tired. Too tired to even imagine another baby. Now I'm wondering: did I wait too long? Are all my eggs gone? My periods are weirder too--lighter, no cramps anymore since my daughter was born. At first, I thought that was a sign of health. Now, I'm guessing it means that my body isn't producing much to give me cramps anymore.

Oh, for the pain of cramps I enjoyed during youth.

How could I have known that those cramps were a sign that my body was toasty and ripe for baby-making?

Sometimes, I see young girls who got pregnant a bit too early and I think: wow, do they know how lucky they are?

By the time they are my age, their children will be 10, 15, sometimes 17 years old. If I had given birth at 18, my child would now be 16 years old.

Imagine...living most of my adulthood with a child to love.

That's how being infertile turns everything on its head. Teenage pregnancy is nothing to envy, but when baby-making becomes the hardest thing in the world to achieve, the ease of a teenager's stroll into babymaking can seem oddly be enviable.

At one time, the idea of having a baby very young seemed like a living prison, a trap to avoid at all costs.

Now it seems ideal.

Had I known what I know now maybe I wouldn't have been so determined to wait.

Wait.

I'm always waiting. I feel like I'm always waiting for something. I'm tired of waiting. I want another baby. Now! I know I am lucky to have my daughter. Without her, I would be in a constant mourning. Because of her, I can bear this.

But as she grows older, I see a certain neediness within her that reminds me of myself. She loves people and when we go out, she immediately wants to connect to other children. The hard part is sometimes other children want to connect and sometimes they don't.

Some children are very friendly, warm and open, and some children are so completely content with their brothers and sisters, they don't want outsiders crashing in and disrupting the status quo.

The bottom line is: I don't feel capable of raising her as an only child, because I don't want to experience a redo of the issues I faced. I loved my childhood, but I want a different experience for her.

It is the same reason that adults from large families who never had their own bedroom or clothes that weren't hand-me-downs have only children: the grass is always greener and we want our children to have what we didn't have.

I want more babies. I need another baby so my daughter won't be lonely. I need a baby so my family will be larger, fuller, noisier. I am craving the commotion that comes with lots of children. I am sad that because of my age, it is unlikely I will ever have the three or four children I once thought I would have.

If I even have one more baby, I am doing well.

Starting Down IVF Road

I had a consultation with Dr. P. today. He says the IUIs don't seem to be working and its time to take the treatments up a notch and move on to IVF. Add to that my age, which is now 37, and the difficulties I encountered getting pregnant the first time, he explained.

So this cycle I will start my first IVF.

Physical Manifestation of My Internal Self

This IVF has been harder than I imagined. It is a dull January. Usually I love winter, but there is nothing cozy-and-hot-chocolately about this winter. I drive constantly to the clinic. I take blood test after blood test. Ultrasound after ultrasound. I'm sick of tests. I'm sick of driving.

Today I went for a routine blood test, and on the way home, a blizzard started. It was snowing wildly, when suddenly, my windshield wipers broke. Just like that, they broke, right on Route 128. I couldn't see a thing. I couldn't even see the road, or the breakdown lane, or anything.

I started praying out loud.

Every few feet, I would roll down the window and put my hand or some object out the window in an attempt to clear the windshield.

The snow was coming down in heaping buckets and most of the drive, I couldn't see a thing.

The whole time I prayed out loud. Please God, let me get home to my daughter. I felt if I could just get home to my daughter, I wouldn't care so much about anything else. Why did I put myself in this danger? Maybe this is a sign that I shouldn't keep trying for a second baby. Maybe I should have been thankful for what I had. Did this happen because I am greedy for trying for another child, when maybe I should just be thankful for what I had?

In two days they remove my eggs. This is not what I need right now--to be on 128 in the middle of a storm and have my windshield wipers break. God, this is so hard right now. I feel desperate, crazy. It is all too much for me.

Finally, I get to an exit and pull off the highway. I had to keep driving to find help, because I don't have a cell phone.

God, I need a cell phone.

The snow falls heavily. I kept driving, until finally I reached a convenience store where I called for help. By the time I reached the store, I was frantic.

I phoned triple AAA and they came and got me.

The whole time, I kept thinking, 'maybe this is what I get for wanting more children--maybe wanting too much is going to be the end of me. Maybe I should have been grateful for what I have."

This incident was a perfect physical manifestation of how alone and in danger I feel lately.

If the physical world can mirror one's inner world, that snapshot of me today, driving down the highway in a blinding snowstorm with no windshield wipers, would be the perfect physical manifestation of my life right now.

This drive seemed like a literal translation of walking by faith, not by sight.I prayed so hard today, as prayer seemed like the only thing I could do.

I remember once a long time ago telling Leah that if I couldn't have babies the natural way, I would just do IVF "they put the egg with the sperm in a dish, and wham, a baby." Wow, was I naive.

Nothing feels fun anymore. I don't like this IVF. It is hard and overwhelming.

First IVF

It is gray today. Everything feels gray. I enter the clinic, and for the first time, I am ushered into the part of the clinic where the IVF patients are sent before they go to the operating room to have their eggs retrieved.

This area in the clinic is deceptively pretty. The wallpaper is a lovely pastel. Once inside, the wallpaper's softness dissolves into an eerie color. This part of the clinic is oddly deserted, compared to the busyness of the rest of the clinic. No one is here, except for one nurse at the check-in.

Since I have done about 17 IUIs, I always imagined that doing an IVF would be no big deal, just another step in my goal to have children. But this is harder than I imagined. I can't say why exactly. Maybe because at this point, I know way too much about baby-making.

I hate waiting in this room, laying so high in this bed, as my daughter runs around.

As sad as the IUIs were, they did not feel quite as heavy as this.

It is scary to be here. Scary to be doing this.

I don't know why I feel so depressed today.

Maybe because the weather is cold and gray and I feel as cold and gray as the weather.

I am the only patient here today, today's sole exhibit in this warped science show.

I need someone to tell me it is going to be all right. It is frightening to think that this seems to be the only way I am going to get a second baby.

The level of stress I am feeling is way too high. No matter how badly I feel right now, it would feel worse not to have the hope of a second baby. So I will endure this gray hell pastel wallpaper and the doctor coming in to tell me that my eggs are poor quality, but that "even poor quality eggs can make a baby" (gee, thanks for the comfort.) Then, later, I will endure learning that out of the ten eggs retrieved today, only three lived. Yikes! What happened to the other seven? I needed those seven. Why did they die? Are my eggs dying because I am too old? Will they all die? Will my other eggs live to make a baby?

I don't like knowing this stuff. I don't like knowing "the quality" of my eggs--or the fact that out of the ten eggs all that medication produced, only three lived to be transferred back into me. Why did those seven eggs die? I was so excited when I learned they retrieved ten eggs. Good for you ovaries, I thought, good job! Man, I thought: seven eggs, of course I'll get a baby out of this. Maybe two or three babies. I kept imagining myself happily exhausted by triplets. My daughter suddenly blessed with three brothers and sisters. Me instantly having the large family of my dreams. Now I know seven eggs have died. I am so sad for those seven eggs. I wanted them to live. Then I'm told my egg quality isn't great. Why isn't my egg quality great? What have I done to make my egg quality so bad? Is it pollution? Bad eating habits? Being fat?

In this part of the hospital, I feel so lonely. It is as if I am being escorted into a life I never wanted. I wanted children younger. I wasn't a CEO of a corporation who chose to wait because I was enjoying some grand career.

Life made me wait, and now I am in this gray zone where baby making isn't a night of lovemaking, but a stilted series of strategic steps that demand I stay on course, disciplined, a pilot at the cockpit during a dangerous storm where one error is not allowed.

One misstep..crash..game over.

Will I ever feel light again? Will anything ever feel easy again?

I am glad science has given me this chance, but I am also sad that I needed science to give me this chance. I am thankful this is not 100 years ago...hell, even 30 years ago, because this chance would not have existed for me. I wish I never had to know the ins and outs of babymaking in the way I know it now—egg quality? Can you imagine anyone in my family ever worrying about their egg quality before? I am the first woman ever in my family, for as far back as time goes, to ever get a baby this way. Ever! In the history of both sides of my family! Thinking about this makes this all seem too serious, too sad and makes me feel too flawed. I want to be 21, in love, in bed, making a baby without thought or strategy or a list of what I need to do today to get pregnant.

I think of women in past generations, trapped because no one could tell them why a baby wasn't coming. I can only imagine the frustration they felt when month after month, no baby came, and there was no ultrasound machines or medications or IVF procedures to give them a chance. At least, despite all this, I have hope and I have options.

After the retrieval, I return to this room, feeling sore and hoping my ovaries were not damaged as they probed me for my eggs. My parents are here to watch my daughter, probably wondering how we all ended up here.

Wasn't I suppose to be a normal girl, who got married and had kids, without all this drama? Somewhere along the way, things in my life got really screwy, and normal things stopped happening. Now, I have to have my Mom and Dad here to watch my daughter while my husband goes to put his sperm in a cup.

My poor eggs.

My poor, poor eggs.

Please God, please. I know that without prayer, I could not
get through this--only my hope that God is helping me enabled me to
keep going today.

Now I have to wait two weeks for the results of this IVF. It has been a
hard few weeks.. all culminating into this one big icky day.

Oops! Pee Pee Problem

The hardest part of the IVF was something I did not expect at all.

It was not the myriad of shots I had to endure every night, or the insane
number of times I had to drive Route 128 during the height of the
morning commute.

It was having to hold my urine after the IVF.

After the eggs and sperm were mixed together and planted back into
me, I was wheeled back to the room and told to hold my urine for a half
an hour.

I did not know that to help the eggs and sperm take hold, they have you
drink an enormous glass of water and hold it.

This sounds simple, right?

Wrong.

It was hard.

So, so hard.

I laid there, dying to just get to a toilet and let it all flow out.

Holding one's pee pee has to be one of the hardest things to do on this earth.

Every part of me was screaming, "Let me go! Let me go! Let me go!"

Nothing in this whole process felt as horrible as being forced to hold an enormous amount of pee. I am expulsive by nature and inherently holding things in--feelings, anything--is grueling and painful.

"How many minutes?" I kept saying to my husband. I'd look at the clock. Five minutes had passed... I wanted to get up and disobey them, but I want this baby so bad...

I stared at the clock: one minute down, five minutes down..ten minutes down. It went so slow.

I hoped that by staring down the clock, the minutes would pass quicker.

Finally, I hit the thirty minute mark. I vaulted out of the bed into the bathroom.

Relief....it never felt so good.

Now I head home and wait for the results to find out if the IVF worked and I am pregnant.

Try, Try Again

I woke up the other morning and knew it had happened.

"I think I got it," I whispered to my husband.

"Oh no," he said softly, in a heavy tone full of sadness.

I tip-toed quietly to the bathroom.

"Yes," I confirmed a few minutes later. "I got it."

The red hot signal that I am not pregnant had arrived.

Inside me, walls came crashing down and others went up.

I should be pregnant. I should be, should
be, should be!

"We'll keep trying for a baby," my husband said kindly.

Try? How dare he! Try was not a word I wanted to hear. The very word 'try' enraged me. Try? Trying isn't an option....we'll make this happen! We'll will it to happen, force it to happen, bend its arm backwards and make it happen.

"What do you mean 'trying'?" I asked him, frustrated that he would relegate having our second child to simply an act of trying and not an act of will.

"I said we'll keep trying," he repeated, not at all understanding why I was getting so mad at him.

The rest of the day was a fuzzy blur. I ended up with a razor sharp headache and a stomache. The next day, I find out that two of my friends are pregnant. They are certainly not specimens of health and yet they are pregnant.

Why is it so easy for some people? Why is it so hard for me?

I need a plan and came up with this:

• My husband will see a nutritionist to strengthen and improve his sperm.

• I will see the same nutritionist.

• I will also go to a person who specializes in emotional release. Sounds flaky, I know, but a friend highly recommends it and for $35 I figure why not try it.

The premise is that trapped emotion in the body can cause illness and dysfunction, and that once negative emotion is released, the body can return to health and normalcy.

My guess is that deep inside me, some sadness is trapped, and perhaps it needs to be released in order for everything in my body to work properly--kind of like an old clock with a big piece of dust preventing the hands from turning.

• I will go to acupuncture once, sometimes twice, a week.

• I will begin eating an extremely healthy diet. I started eating healthier a few months ago, and recently I have seen a big increase in the number of eggs I am producing.

• I will also swim everyday, or every other day. Swimming for me is a great stress reliever.

• I will pray more, although I already pray about 1,000 times a day. Prayer is a privilege that I cannot imagine living without. Thank God that He gave us the ability to talk to Him and go to Him for help. I will ask God to show me what I need to do in order to heal my body and conceive a second child.

Getting Happier

Today I had an appointment with Dr. Deutsch and Eileen. I started going to them to help me clear out past traumas and bad memories, as a way to free up energy in my body to get pregnant. Leah goes to them and recommended I start going, just to clear out anything from my past that might still be lodged in my body. Thankfully, I listened to her and they have turned out to be more than amazing.

I see them every Tuesday. It is an hour and a half trip, but so worth it.

Dr. Deutsch is a chiropractor and an expert in kinesiology. Eileen does myofascial release. Eileen has been working on helping me release sad memories from the past that have been weighing me for years.

Sometimes, it is small things—a hurt from a childhood friend that happened 20+ years ago. A teenage break-up. The body seems to hold everything. I give her a list of names, and it is surprising to find who has smudged their emotional fingerprint on me and who hasn't.

She explained that she is preparing my body to receive.

Sometimes during the treatments I cry a little. Afterward, I feel relief. I feel lighter and lighter, like the joyous 18 year old girl I once was is being resurrected.

After Eileen works on me, Dr. Deutsch follows up. Today, I released so much emotion, when Dr. Deutsch came into the room, he started waving his hand and fanning himself, as if, wow a lot of emotional energy has been released today.

On the way home, I felt overcome with a rush of pure happiness. The sun was shining, a Maine country radio station was playing, and I was feeling lighter than I've felt in years

I am spending a load of money on this right now--about $140 every time I go to them. I'm not buying any clothes. We don't have a second car, and the $400 our tenant Lenny pays us is primarily used for these treatments.

I am lucky to have found this new way of healing.

With Eileen and Dr. Deutsch, I am experiencing a transformation I never imagined possible. Things that hurt or bothered me for 20 years all of a sudden don't bother me anymore.

I never imagined that much of the emotional pain living inside me could be erased, like an eraser on a chalkboard. I never understood that the body stores emotional pain in a physical way...and it can be removed!

That is why something that happened at age 5 can feel as fresh and raw as the day it happened 40 years later.

It can sound hocus-pocus when you learn about this for the first time, but it isn't.

When I see Eileen, it is as if she is vacuuming my body clean of all emotional pain.

Driving home today, I felt like I used to feel back in college--light, hopeful, full of optimism.

I have not felt like this for a very long time.

Truthfully, it is a feeling I thought would never return.

Sometimes in life, you experience things that are so painful, you enter a place so dark, that even when you finally escape the darkness, parts of you stay prisoner of that darkness—and the light never shines through to you as fully as it once did.

Now, because of Eileen and Dr. Deutsch, I won't have to live my entire life filled with long-ago wounds.

A ride home on 95 South, sun-a-shining/radio-a-blaring/the new-me-old-me-new-me emerging. Times are a changing.

Writing My Life Story and Seeing Patterns

Next week is my appointment with Begbetti, a homeopathic expert in Cambridge, MA.

She mailed me a questionnaire and asked me to write my life story, that will help her determine what patterns in my life need to be unblocked.

Writing this life story has been revealing. It seems my life has two themes running simultaneously: one is about joy, happiness, friendship, achievement and faith. The other theme is loss and rejection.

I wrote about losing my best friend in seventh grade to the 'cool kids' and this pattern of loss, followed by great mourning and sadness, seems to be a reoccurring theme in my life.

There seems to be a lot of dramatic endings in my relationships. It was hard to write this and see in black-and-white all my failures.

I'm bringing a copy of my life story to Eileen so she can work on helping me to release some these memories. I know all these painful losses live inside me and are sapping physical strength from me.

How can I successfully carry a baby for nine months, when I carry around so many lost people in my heart?

First Homeopathy Appointment

Today was my first appointment with Beghbetti. It started snowing on my way there and of course, (no surprise) my windshield wipers broke. Why do they only break when I am doing something to help me get pregnant?

I couldn't drive without wipers, but I was not about to miss this appointment, so I called Triple AAA and had them tow me and my car to a parking spot near her office.

I'll deal with getting home later.

Beghbetti's office hip, warm earthy,and welcoming.

She asked me lots of questions, like: do I like to sleep with the window closed or open? What type of things am I afraid of. Then she prescribed a remedy for me.

Tonight, I took the remedy for the first time. The moment I finished swallowing it, I felt a sharp pain jump out of my left breast and a throbbing pain leave my right buttock.

I have no idea why that happened, but I'm hoping something is changing in my body.

I'm glad I didn't let the broken wiper stop me from getting to my appointment.

Needing People to Talk To

Every day, no matter what I am doing, all I think about is whether or not I will ever be able to give my daughter a brother or a sister.

No matter where we are or how much fun we are having, the thought of getting pregnant is always scampering around my head.

Infertility is a part of everything I do, twining itself around every experience I have, whether I like it or not.

For example, on Monday, my mother and I went to the mall for ice cream and a friend who also went to the same fertility clinic as I did works in the food court.

I saw him and his wife at the clinic the day I had my laparoscopy and was being wheeled down to the operating room, when the elevator doors opened and Tom and his wife walked in.

It was a pretty incredible coincidence. Neither one of us knew that the other was going through infertility treatments.

Then, today we found out Tom is one of the managers at the ice cream place at the mall where we get my daughter her Monday cup of vanilla ice cream as part of our routine.

Now every Monday, I get to see Tom and guess what I talk about? It feels so good to talk to someone who knows the same doctors I do, whose has sat with his wife through the same tests I've endured, and who even can talk about which medications worked best for them.

It is a wonderful part of my week, because with Tom, I am comfortable enough to burp up my worries, even if just for a few minutes.

I usually ask Tom questions, but really what I'm looking for is hope, reassurance, words from someone who believes it will all work out for me.

Tom is very comforting. Not only is he a nice person who offers simple but positive comments like "it will all work out. Don't worry," but he has experienced the success of having infertility treatments culminate into the birth of his daughter last year.

He is the only person I know, other than my husband, who can understand the world I inhabit when I walk in that clinic.

We've exchanged opinions about which doctors have the best bedside manner, which ones answer questions the best, and which ones administer tests with the least amount of pain.

Overall, I don't talk much about my infertility this second-time around. Sharing my feelings with most people is not very comforting, but usually makes me just panic more. I see in the faces of those around me fear and an expectation of disappointment. They are afraid to see me hurt again. They think by not giving me hope they are shielding me from falling too far down if this doesn't work out. I feel more and more like I am cast off on a lonely island. I have to live inside my own head right now. I can't face hearing out loud from another person the possibility that my daughter will never have a biological sibling. As I write these words, I almost fall apart. It can't happen. I won't let it.

 I'm not asking for a lot--just one more sibling--not five, not four, not even three, just one right now. As much as I enjoy every minute with my daughter, there is a constant gray cloud hanging over me, a threat that our family will never be larger than it is right now, a family with two adults and one child.

Sometimes when we go to the park, and there are siblings playing together, and my daughter is trying to break in, my heart tumbles in defeat.

What she doesn't understand is that she can't break in to what they have, no matter how much she tries. When I see her so wanting to be friends with every child she meets, there is nothing I desire more than to give her a sibling who will be her friend, and who will shield her from at the mercy of childhood friendships' that can be fickle in nature.

There are a few people I still talk to: my mother, Leah, Tom and Judy. If I see even a glimmer of fear or anxiety on their face, I fall apart. It is better I keep this all in my own head right now. I can lie to myself very well. I can keep hope alive. I can ignore even the most basic tenets of reality when I have to.

I'm relying on my faith in God right now, on my belief in miracles and the body's ability to heal. I believe the impossible is possible. Alone without other voices, I can hold on to this way of thinking without interruption.

I believe God opened the Red Sea when all looked hopeless.
I believe he heard the cries of Hannah who desperately wanted a child. I believe that scripture that says if you have faith, you can say to a mountain move this way or move that way, and it will move. If I didn't believe this way, I would give up right now, because a lot of evidence is against me and the physical world does not seem to be supporting my dream. Instead, I have entered a reality of believing without physical evidence. Faith is all I have.

So I just keep praying and staying silent.

I am anxious for it all to work out.

NOT MUCH IMPROVEMENT! Are you kidding me?

Today I felt lousy all the way around. I went to Dr. Kim for acupuncture and asked him how my body was doing. I expected to hear some glowing report on how much progress I made. Instead, he felt my pulse, frowned a bit, and said frankly, my life force was still weak.

Still weak?

I have been going to acupuncture every week for almost three months and I am still weak?

'Not much improvement," he repeated.

Come on! I didn't need to hear that!

After that comment, I felt pretty lousy the rest of the day. All day at work, I kept thinking: why isn't my body getting better? I have to shake what he said out of my head. Isn't even a bit of an improvement still an improvement? I can't help but worry.

Praying Hard

Prayer is an integral part of my infertility treatments. God is my partner in this infertility quest.

I don't pray expecting that if I make all the wrong choices, I'll still get a baby. I pray that He gives me the strength to keep trying when I want to give up. I pray that He helps me find the right doctors and do the right things to heal my body.

I don't naively think if I pray for a baby, but drink sugary soda, miss important appointments, keep on this extra weight, and guzzle coffee that my body is going to produce the baby of my dreams. I know God hears my prayers and I know He wants good things for me, but I also believe He has gifted me with power over my life to some degree. I have the power to make choices, to investigate information and pursue treatments that will help me.

So I don't just pray to have a baby, but I also pray to find the right treatments to heal my infertility.

I read that when you have a goal, you have to be ready to walk through fire to attain the goal.

Well, I'm ready. I would cut off my foot if it guaranteed that I would have a baby. I will go anywhere, spend any amount of money I have, try just about anything to make my body able to conceive and give birth.

I have to work along with my prayers, and if my prayer is for a baby, I have to be doing things to get myself healthy enough to have a baby.

I think the biggest lie told about God is that He wants to deny humans and say no to their requests whenever possible.

I can't say how many people have said right out loud, or insinuated, that God may not want me to have a second baby. Why do so many people naturally and easily assume that if I want a second baby, God doesn't want me to have one? Why do they find it so easy to think God wants to deny me what I most want? Why can't they think that God wants good things for me--and why wouldn't a second baby be good for me? Why is everyone so ready to attribute everything bad or denied in their life to God saying no, when really it could be their own choices, their own lack of initiative and willpower, or their own choice to stay a victim rather than work hard to improve the situation?

If I give up now, should I blame God if I never have a second child--or blame myself for giving up?

Maybe God wants me to have a baby, but He is leaving it up to me to keep trying.

I do not blame God for my infertility. I blame human imperfection. I am sick. I am not ashamed that I have infertility problems. I am tired of people insinuating there is something shameful about my condition.

I am not ashamed.

I am not a bad person because I have problems getting pregnant.

I am not a weak person, a morally bad person, a cursed person, or a woman punished by God.

I am not weird and do not deserved to be whispered about because of my problem.

I am a person with a health problem, who is seeking to get healthier and who is asking God to help me.

I do not pray and eat Twinkies.

I do not pray and do nothing. That would be an insult to the power God has given me over my life.

I have choices. I have the ability to seek out answers to the questions in my life, and right now, the question is: why is my body having trouble getting pregnant?

I think God wants me to have another baby. I think He wants my daughter to have a sibling to love. I think He will help me. I think He also expects me to work hard for this myself. I do not assume He will say no just because I want to hear a yes.

On Track Like Never Before

I don't think there has ever been a time in my life when I have been more focused, more with my eye on the ball, than I am right now.

When I wake up every day, the first question on my mind is: what can I do today to get one step closer to being pregnant? Then I write in my daily appointment book what I can do to help me reach my goal.

I can't do an IVF for another two months. During that time, I'll whatever I can to get healthy: bowls of romaine lettuce, chicory and parsley, which everyone at work jokes as being my "rabbit food."

I juice spinach, snack on walnuts, and have cut out most white flour and sugar products. When I think of how I used to eat--lots of cheese and meat, so much bread and white flour, I am amazed that my body was able to take it. My head actually feels like it is clearing a bit on this new diet. I sometimes joke that I'm taking a kamikaze approach to healing. Or maybe it's a 'if-you-throw-enough-darts-you'll-eventually-hit-the-target' approach. Basically, I'll try anything that seems remotely reasonable to get my body strong enough to have a baby.

Every day, I vascillate wildly on the hope meter. I'm up! I'm down.... I'm optimistic! I crash....

One moment, I am having fun with my daughter and loving my life. A moment later, I see her bored, lonely, wanting to play with other children, and a fingernail-on-the-chalkboard desperation to get pregnant hits me.

For the first time in my life, I understand the power of looking at a problem from every angle, and the power of making good choices. Maybe, for the first time, I see clearly my role in how this will all turn out.

As sad as I sometimes feel, I don't think I've ever been more on top of a situation than I am right now.

Does Loss of Authentic Personality Equals Loss of Fertility?

Today was my first appointment with Dr. Zhu, an acupuncturist and master herbalist, who I wanted to try because I've heard a lot of wonderful things about Chinese herbs helping infertility.

I have to say that driving to his office was among the worst driving experiences I've had lately. But then, driving to the clinic is pretty harrowing too. I have no choice but to drive this highway, but sometimes I feel like the drive down Route 128 is a metaphor for my infertility: you must do what you have to do to get to your destination, regardless of how frightening and horrifying it feels.

Dr. Zhu's office was so peaceful, in contrast to my drive over. He felt my pulse, which acupuncturists and Chinese herbalists do to determine what is wrong. He then had me read a paragraph from a book on what he considered to be some of my problems. The paragraph described me perfectly.

Then he put together a bag of herbs for me to boil and make into a tea.

Before I left, he gave me a short, but very powerful, acupuncture treatment. During Dr. Khu's treatment, I could actually feel parts of my brain opening that had been closed off for a long time.

After he inserted the needles, I sat reading a 'People' magazine article about the problem of bullying in the school systems, and how one young boy even committed suicide because he was so tormented by bullies. I was overwhelmed with inspiration, got out my notebook and started jotting down ideas how to curb the bullying problem.

In all, I wrote nine pages on how to stop bullying and while I wrote, I felt different than I had in a long time: powerful and capable of changing things, unblocked by the usual shame, fear, embarrassment or failure I often feel when I imagine that I can change things. It was like an old part of me resurfaced that wasn't ashamed or burdened down with memories of failures.

Charging forward with solutions and fighting for causes was a part of who I was long time ago. Over time, and with lots of failures, I lost this part of me who believed I could change things or make things better for others. When I was a child, I was always coming up with ideas to fix things and right wrongs. I ran a Jerry Lewis carnival for muscular dystrophy, got signatures for a Save the Whales petition, and in college organized a two-week Feed the World weeks festival, where the governor of Massachusetts declared April 25 Feed the World Day.

'Feed the World' weeks turned out to be a big disaster. I was 19 and not really ready to undertake a fundraising operation of this size. We raised $5,000, but I made a million mistakes. The experience shrank me. After that, I never had the confidence to spearhead anything again. When I heard about this crisis or that crisis, I no longer imagined that I could do something about it.

Maybe I lost the belief that I was competent enough to make positive change. I never consciously realized, or even acknowledged, that this change had come over me, but my life slowly became more about protecting, hiding and defending myself, rather than reaching out to help and make a difference.

Yet, all of a sudden during this treatment, I felt that activist part of me come back to life. I felt angrily energized about the problem of bullying in America and I somehow felt capable of coming up with solutions to the problem, much the way I used to feel when I was young.

Is it possible that this acupuncture treatment resurrected a dead part of me that was once a pillar of my personality? And how did losing this part of me relate to my infertility?

Is my infertility related to an inability to manifest my will and power in this world?

What is the correlation between my infertility and this loss in my personality?

I can't speculate too much about this--as I don't really know what this treatment did to me exactly, but I wonder if the disappearance of who I am also weakened my body's ability to manifest things I care about in general.

I left very contented to have added yet another layer to my healing.

Second Homeopathic Treatment

Today, I had my second visit with Begbetti.

What a sharp contrast to my first visit. The first time I went there, I felt very stressed—like the elements were against me and yet another snow storm was trying to block me from getting the treatments I needed.

This time, it was a beautiful spring day. As I walked up the Cambridge side street to her office, I felt an old buoyancy return that I haven't felt in years.
I felt light-hearted, dare I say happy even, in a way I haven't felt since college.

Way back in college, before I had my heart broken about 100 times, before I had lost jobs at places I thought I would work at forever, before I failed at so many things, I walked around with a kind of happy, confident, naive girl-in-white optimism.

Youth, some people would call it.

 I have always longed to regain that feeling--a feeling that life is beautiful and great things were within my reach. I struggled many times to get back to the me that was capable of enjoying the quiet of nature on a beautiful day. As hard as I tried, I could not get back to that whole, happy me.

Beauty in nature made me sad, uncomfortable, because my insides no longer matched the beauty of the outdoor world.

Today, surrounded by the dizzying beauty of spring, I felt the old me return.

Beghbetti's receptionist, Paris, noticed the change in me right away. "You seem so much happier than you did the first time you came here," she said. "You look so alive."

Perhaps everything I am doing to heal: going to Eileen, Dr. Deutsch, Dr. Kim and Dr. Zhu, is healing something deep inside me and restoring parts of me that I thought were lost forever.

At today's appointment, Beghbetti asked me more questions, like what type of weather conditions I feel most comfortable in. I told her I like the winter a lot, but hot summer weather seems to bring up anger and a sense of helplessness in me. She prescribed a remedy.

I left feeling full of hope. This healing process to get pregnant has turned out to be exactly what I needed on many levels, aside from just the infertility aspect. I have been in emotional pain for a long time. So many heavy hurts were trapped inside me, and now I have been given a chance to heal and remove them permanently.

My Diet Is Actually Working

My diet is actually working and I am actually losing weight. People are noticing. For the first time in ten years, a diet has worked.

My motivation to look better is about stabilizing my hormones to increase my chance of getting pregnant.

I hit my highest weight about a year after my daughter was born. I went on this pepper-steak-onion-cheddar-cheese-in-a-wrap binge, and one can imagine how I looked after eating those night after night.

Now I eat foods I once wouldn't have dreamed of eating and it is amazing how much more energy I have.

When I got married nine years ago, I was tired by 1 in the afternoon and would sometimes spend the rest of the day in bed watching TV. Now, I can go all day, and still have energy left at night.

This whole infertility ordeal has changed all sorts of patterns in my life. It has forced me to become a disciplined soldier in this war I'm waging against all the forces conspiring to keep me without the family I long for. This includes my own self-destructive habits and my own self-hatred that often thinks that I should end up alone and with nothing.

Sometimes, when I listen to the theme from Rocky, I envision myself in a jungle, climbing and swinging through trees with my daughter strapped to my back. It is for her I am trudging through this jungle of infertility. For her, I will climb trees and fight lions and paddle down raging rivers.

For every nasty, uncomfortable, painful test I have to endure, the image of my daughter enjoying a sibling keeps me going.

It is amazing what one a person can do when there is enough desire.

I have not been able to lose weight in years, but now when I am tempted to buy a candy bar in the vending machine at work, I say to myself: 'that candy bar could prevent you from ever having another baby' and suddenly I can reject even chocolate! I lived for a long time through a weaker version of myself, a version that wanted to hide, and didn't want to try too hard for anything because she was too sad and scared. I was tired all the time and just wanted to rest from all the sad experiences I had. Now I will do whatever it takes. My family will not be complete until we have another child. He or she has to come to us—or our family will have a gaping hole in it.

Infertility is testing me and pushing me, and I like the person I am becoming because of it.

Back to the Clinic

Awhile back, I decided to change doctors. I left Dr. P and switched to Dr. M, a female doctor, because I need a change. I am so worn out emotionally right now, that I need some kind of a change. I need a doctor with more of a bedside manner. Each time I had to see Dr. P after hearing some bad or disappointing news, he acts like it is the most inconsequential of events. I realize he must deal with hundreds of people every month, and he has a basic kindness that comes through, but I don't have the strength for so much logic and rational right now. I need a bit more babying, and since Dr. M was so kind during some of the tests she administered, I wanted to try her.

Good thing I did.

She immediately discovered from an ultrasound taken this morning that I have a large fibroid that needs to be removed.

A fibroid! That explains everything! I am thrilled at this news!

Finally, I know why I am not getting pregnant.

I feel so relieved right now. Once the fibroid is out, I'll be able to get pregnant and have another baby in no time!

Maybe this has been my problem all along. When did this fibroid start? Before my daughter was born? After my daughter was born? Thank God this fibroid didn't hurt my daughter. I hate it intensely. And how did it get so big?

I am so glad that at least now, I have a clear and true explanation for my fertililty problems.

My Most Private Journals: What My Subconscious Had To Say

Here's a peek at the journals I wrote from the point of view of my subconscious as I tried to dig out what my subconscious self was truly feeling and experiencing at this time.

Journal 1

Me: I am having a baby.

Subconscious: A baby--you? You big loser? You know what a loser you are. A baby? You couldn't have a pet cat if you tried. (Note: today I have four pets cats so I guess my subconscious was very wrong!) A baby--oh my God, everyone knows you are too old and too worn out. You can't handle anything. Do you realize what a screw up you are? Paula, the road to hell is paved with good intentions, and you are that road to hell. I can't believe you think this can work out. Get a grip.

Me: I am having a baby. I am having a healthy beautiful baby. I am pregnant right now.

Subconscious: Oh God, you are nothing. I can't believe you buy this optimism crap. I think you better give up my dear, because you are worthless.

Me: My vagina is strong and my baby is growing healthy inside me. I can carry a baby.

Subconscious: You can't carry a baby. Hasn't it been proven your eggs are too old and too messed up? You have some problem--maybe mercury, but give up weirdo. You are indeed a big weirdo. You are not like all the other women who had babies young. You are too old. You are very old.

Me: I am pregnant and in nine months I'm going to have a baby.

Subconscious: Wishful thinking. You are meant to struggle and get nothing. You are meant to be perpetually punished for your sins. No one ever believes in you.

Me: I like myself. I believe I can have more babies. I am strong. I make good eggs.

Subconscious: Stop the bravado. It isn't working on me. I feel like you can't have any more kids. Dr. M said you were too old--and I believe her. You look old. You feel old. You seem like the world has gone by you on this one. God hates you too. How could He like you? How in the world could you think God would help you?

Me: I can have babies. I am having more babies. My body is creating more babies.

Subconscious: Your friend had a baby with one ovary, barely made any eggs, and somehow got a baby out of the deal, a nice boy baby. You are not looking for gold--you want one more baby. You can do this. Look, it may be hard. It may be a long road. No one said this will be easy. You need help along the way. But ultimately, you can have a baby. You won't do stupid things. You'll rest a lot. You'll go to Eileen and Dr. Deutsch a lot. You'll get help.

Journal 2: I ask my body why it was having trouble getting pregnant.

Me: Why can't I have a baby?

Subconscious: Because you are bad. Because you are not worth anything. Because you get envious and anxious and something is wrong with you. Because you are not worth anything. Because you deserve nothing

Me: Why can't I have another baby?

Subconscious: Because you only get one shot at happiness. Because you can't escape your fate.

Me: I hate my life. I am stuck. I am in a hole. I am disappearing. I'm tired of people telling me to give up and accept. I am never giving up! That is not me. I am not giving up at all. I never give up when I want something. I want a second baby. No! I want ten babies. Two is not enough. I want many, many, many, babies. Give me more babies! Give me more!

Subconscious: No! You are a bad girl. Other girls will get everything-- you get nothing. You are a loser. You can't escape your life. You are a weirdo. A loser.

Journal 3: I wrote this when I was pregnant with my son.

Me: I am going to have a second baby in nine months.

Subconscious: Bull! Nothing ever goes right for you.

You are a big loser. You always have bad things happen to you. That is your lot in your life. You try and try and get nothing. Everyone sees you as a loser. Everyone still sees you as that girl who can't get anything she wants. Why would this be different?

Me: Shut up! You are wrong. I am having this baby. For your information, people believe in me. I am not a messed up. I am a strong woman. A good mother. I am a determined person. I have worked hard to earn this baby. I have gone through test after test, shot after shot. I earned this baby and I'm going to see my reward.

Subconscious: How? How are you going to see it?

Me: Because I am a strong person. Because my body is strong. Because this time, I am arming myself. Because God is on my side. Because my vagina is strong, my uterus is strong, and I love my baby. I love this little baby inside of me. I adore him. I love him. He is already my best friend.

This child will be my daughter's best friend. They will play house together and love each other. She will have a readymade support system.

She will have what other people have: a built in network of people to love. When we go to weddings, my daughter will have a companion, she will not be at the mercy of bratty children who ignore her.

Subconscious: Honey, I see you are sad. You are such a wonderful girl. You will have your own babies.

Journal 4: I ask my body what it needs.

Me: Okay vagina and uterus, talk. Tell me what you are feeling.

Subconscious: I am feeling helpless. I am not feeling loved. I want to hear 'Rocky.' Do you understand what I've gone through? It is hard on me. (Note: it is a good idea to ask your subconscious what it needs. There might be something this part of you needs that it is not getting, or a deep need that is being ignored)

Me: What do you need?

Subconscious: Bring me an afghan. Bring me peace. Bring me time in the Arctic with penguins. Bring me good books. Bring me love. Bring me Rona Jaffe. *(Note that my subconscious gives specifics as to what she needs and in knowing this, I can help calm her down and comfort her.)*

Journal 5: Note some of the self-hatred that I had to work through in order to feel worthy of receiving my goal.

Me: I want a second baby.

Subconscious: No you don't. Only young women deserve babies.

You are too old. You can't have it all-your fun and then all the children. You can't get everything in this world. You need to choose either one or the other.

Me: I want a baby.

Subconscious: So what? Lots of people want things they can't get. What makes you any different? Aren't you the same as everybody else?

Me: I deserve to have a baby.

Subconscious: Nope, sorry. Only good girls get babies. You ruined your liver kidney channel. You deserve nothing.

Me: I am going to have a baby.

Subconscious: Nope. Sorry. the answer is no. You don't want a baby deep down. To start all over again--oh Lord no. I can't go through that again. I can't go through the scare of the nine months, the delivery, the horrible recovery, the bleeding, the stitches, the whole thing is too much for me.

Let my body alone--we are tired and we try too hard. (Note that my subconscious is expressing its fatigue and fear of going through another pregnancy. Because I knew that, I knew I had to give myself the rest and security I deserved throughout this pregnancy.)

Me: I am going to have a baby.

Subconscious: Nope, your eggs are old. You used them up. That is what you get.

Me: I am going to have a baby. *(Note: I repeated my wish over and over, as a way to bring up from the subconscious conflicts and to bring my subsconscious over to my conscious side.)*

Subconscious: No, sorry. You deserve nothing. The baby thing is over and done with. Forget it. Don't drive yourself crazy. Enjoy your daughter and forget about it. No one listens to you. No one believes in you. I don't want to go through invitro again. I don't want to have to put under, and have my legs opened up, and to have to hold my urine for seven minutes--they are going to kill me with that. My bladder can't take it. It is too hard. I am too tired for this.

Me: I am going to have a baby.

Journal 6

Me: I am going to have a baby.

Subconscious: No goofhead--you are going to have heartache. You are going to cry. You are a big nobody who nobody loves. You are a loser. Your husband is going to leave you. I wish you would just give up. I am tired of doing stuff, tired of trying. Does it really matter?
You are never going to be happy anyways. You are a loser. Everyone knows that. You are a big loser. You are never going to change. You are a joke. I think you are a weasel. Everyone sees through you. Nobody actually likes you.

Me: I am going to be pregnant soon and have a baby.

Subconscious: A baby? No way! You are alone now and will always be alone. You are a weirdo and you've never been able to hold on to any relationship.

Me: I am going to get pregnant and have a baby. I am strong and my body can do this. I have good eggs inside of me.

Subconscious: No way! You heard Dr. M--you are bottom of the barrel. It is a joke. Why do you keep doing this? Putting yourself through this? You are a glutton for punishment. Paula Paula--the girl who works hard for nothing. The girl who keeps going even when she should give up. Why do you make everything so hard for me? Why do you keep me working and working for nothing? You are always out there, chipping away, doing too much. I feel sorry for you.

Me: I am going to get pregnant soon. Then I'm going to have a beautiful pregnancy and have a baby soon.

Subconscious: You--a beautiful pregnancy! Honey, nothing ever goes that smoothly for you.

You are not the type to enjoy that much smoothness. For you, life is one big down hill rollercoaster ride. Other people get good stuff--you just try and have a good heart, but can't really pull it together. You keep trying, old good hearted one, your efforts are nice, but you can't get results.

Me: I am going to get pregnant soon. I am going to have a healthy, beautiful pregnancy and then give birth to a healthy baby. I am going to enjoy this whole process.

Subconscious: Maybe. Remember: you are a big loser.

Me: I am going to get pregnant soon. I am going to have a healthy, beautiful, safe pregnancy, then I'm going to give birth to a healthy baby.

Subconscious: You are going to have a sick, damaged baby. You are going to have a weird deformed baby. You are a weirdo dear.

Me: I am going to get pregnant soon. I am going to have a healthy baby, and a beautiful, safe pregnancy.

Subconscious: Only young girls can have healthy babies. You were different and weird to begin with, and you'll always be different and weird.

Me: I am going to get pregnant soon. I am going to have a healthy, safe, beautiful pregnancy. I am going to have a healthy baby.

Subconscious: How in the world are you going to do that? You are almost 37 years old---3 years from 40. You are no spring chicken. How would this happen? Do you think your old body can really do this? You are a stressed out, unhappy, overworked and underpaid girl.

Me: I feel so tired. I can't possibly keep going. I am so so discouraged inside of myself. I am so so so tired. I am beyond tired. I want to stop, get on my knees, got to the water and swim. I can't keep going.

Will I ever get peace in my life? When will peace come to me? I have no idea when peace will come? I dream of having a life I want.
I am willing to work for it, but I'm so tired. I am so emotionally tired.

I am tired of dealing with jerks and prickheads. I am tired of dealing with stupid people. I am tired of the subtle rejections and hurt feelings all around me.

Journal 7

Me: I am pregnant.

Subconscious: No ! You? You who mess up everything. I can't be pregnant. I'm afraid to be pregnant. So much can go wrong. I'm going to scream. What if I miscarry? My husband will kill me. I can't take this. I can't take the nine long months. I want the baby here now. I want the baby here right now. I can't wait. I need to see the baby, touch the baby, feel the baby. I need to grow a baby. Oh God, I am not up to this. I am a delicate little flower who wilts in the sun and wind. I am not strong enough to have a baby. I am not tough enough. I am just a woman. A small woman. A frail woman. I'm a woman who tries hard and who messes up and doesn't seem to be the right kind of woman. I am a messed up woman. I am so messed up. I hate myself. I hate everything.

Me: I am going to have a baby. Maybe two or three babies.

Subconscious: Everyone will hurt you. You are the mercy of everyone. You will end up being hurt. You always start out on the right foot and end up goofing up. It is amazing you even have one child. Why should you have more than one beautiful baby when some people get nothing?

You deserve nothing. *(Note a deeply held belief I needed to heal from and overcome.)*

Me: I am going to have a baby. My babies are growing strong.

Subconscious: The stress is too much for me. What if something goes wrong? I can't bare to disappoint anyone. I am just one person. I don't want to disappoint anyone. I want this to work out. I am going to scream. I need to see Eileen every single day. I need to see Dr. Deutsch every single day. I need to do too many things. I need to scream and yell, and scream and yell some more.

Me: I am going to have a baby. Maybe two or three babies. I am a strong mother. I am a very strong woman. No one perseveres like me. *(Note that I continue to speak positively as a way to counteract the negative emotions of my subconscious.)*

Subconscious: Oh God, I'm so afraid. Please God, let this pregnancy be normal, safe, happy, noneventful. Let the time pass quickly. Let it fly by. Let my baby be okay. Please God, Help me, without your help, nothing can work out. What if God hates me? God must hate me. Why would He love me? Why in the world would God love me? What have I ever done to have God love me? If anything, God must hate me. I must be hated. I deserve to be hated. I am a hateful person. I am an evil person. I deserve only bad things to happen to me. I am a bad woman.

Me: I am going to have a baby. My body is strong. I eat good, I exercise, I take my vitamins. I walk, I sing, I dance, I think positive thoughts. I need to keep going. I need to pray constantly. How will I live? How will I keep going? How will I not think about the baby inside me? I am so stressed out being pregnant. So much pain around being pregnant. I can't take all the pain. I can't take all the possibilities in my life right now. What if they all end up being nothing? What if they end up being one big mess up? What if I lose all my chances? I'm right at the door of everything I want. Will I go in that door?

Me: Yes! Yes! Yes! I will walk in that door. No one and nothing will stop me from walking through that door of joy. I've been here before, and I never realized that I deserve--yes really deserve--to walk in this door. I'm doing good things. I'm giving my daughter siblings. When she is old, she can go food shopping with her siblings.

When she comes home from school, she'll have a pal to talk with, laugh with, play with, and be there if friends hurt her. No way! My daughter will have someone to love. She will have someone to play with. She will have someone who invites her over on special days off, someone who will love her and hopefully watch out for her like I do.

Me: (continued) I deserve this! I'm a good person. I deserve this! I deserve joy. I've wasted so much time in sadness, and it got me nowhere. I want the joy. I want the happiness. I want the good stuff. (Note that once I express my negative self-doubts, I am then able to move on to feelings of worth.)

I want all the good stuff I can get. I am ready to get. I'm tired of always waiting for good stuff to happen. I deserve good things. I am a good person. I deserve good things. I worked very hard for this. I sacrificed, I kept going, I spend money, I didn't stop. A big screw you to anyone who wants to take this from me.

Subconscious: I am anxious. I want it all now. I want my baby now. The journey, thus far, was easier when I wasn't so near everything. Now I'm near to getting everything and I'm incredibly scared and incredibly nervous. It is scary to come so close to having everything you want. Oh God, what am I going to do? How am I going to do this? What if I kill myself in the process?

Me: I am going to have a baby. My baby inside of me are growing strong and healthy.

Subconscious: You Paula couldn't grow a cucumber big and strong. You are a big loser. You are not an earthy Mama. You are not a fertility queen. You are not a baby producer. You are a dried up little nerd. You are different than other woman.

You are not allowed to be like other women. You are bad to want a baby. You don't need or deserve two or three babies. You deserve nothing. You are nothing.

Me: I am going to have babies. There are babies--beautiful babies-- growing inside of me--strong and healthy. Yay! I deserve this! I'm a servant of God. God loves me. God answers my prayers.
God knows my heart. God is helping me.

Subconscious: God doesn't want you to have babies. How could you do this? Are you sure God wants more babies in this world? You are a selfish person. What a selfish prick you are. You are ordinary.

You are a selfish lady Paula. Who are you going to help now?

How are you going to help save mankind? You deserve nothing. You deserve to suffer. I hate you so much--that is what you deserve. You think things are so easy. I say that you are a weirdo and you deserve nothing in this world.

I would like to see you suffer some more. I would like to see you miscarry just to prove what a bad person you are. I hate you. I want to see only bad for you. You deserve nothing in this world.

You were and are a bad person. God only blesses good people and you are not one of those good people. Do you understand? I hate you. I hate you so much. (*Note how my subconscious sees only negatives for me, but as she speaks, she begins to express her need for help.*) I am stressed! Help me! God, help me! Get me through this time! I am going to scream! I am trying to escape, wishing I was somewhere else. The journey is so long, and I beg for help. I cannot be sent back there. I need to stop thinking.

Me: I am going to have two or three babies. My babies are growing strong. They are nice babies. They are kind babies. They are good babies. They will make the earth a better place. My daughter's life is going to be better. I am a strong mother. I am a wise mother. I am a woman who is ripe for baby-making. Wow--I am a baby making machine.

Subconscious: You can't do this.

Me: Yes I can.

Subconscious: No you can't.

Me: Yes, I can!

Journal 8

Me: I am having a baby.

Subconscious: No! You don't deserve a baby. You are no good. Remember how nothing you were? Remember how completely horrible you were? Remember? You don't deserve everything. You have to suffer for the rest of your life for your sins. Do you think you can just have so much fun? Good people deserve to have working vaginas and working ovaries. You are all dried up now, a curse from God above for your sins. You are an ugly, nondeserving, stupid person. You are nothing. I won't let you have a baby because I don't think you deserve it.

I think you need to suffer more. You need to suffer and suffer and suffer. I hate the life you created for me. This isn't what I wanted.

I want respect. I want love. I want quiet peace. Nothing went right for me. Everything that could have gone wrong went wrong. I'm so tired of trying for things. A baby? Why--so one day I can wake up and be bleeding. Does anyone understand how much I have lost?

Me: I am having a baby.

Subconscious: Why? Why do you want a baby. I don't want a baby. I want to go to Channel 2. I don't want to go through all the hell I've gone through. I am ugly. I can't take nothing happening anymore. I can't take any more disappointment. I need this to work. (Note that my subconscious enjoys work and doesn't want to miss work due to a pregnancy—acknowledging this is a step towards resolving inner conflict and setting up situations that work for all parts of me.)

Me: I am having a baby.

Subconscious: You? You loser of the year. You having a baby? No one thinks you can have a baby. Everyone knows you are a nice goodhearted person who simply will never get anything. Everyone knows that.

Special people who deserve everything are the ones who get the babies, not you. You are the weird girl. You are a loser, a weirdo.

Me: I am having a baby.

Subconscious: Yah--and do you think your vagina is strong enough to hold a baby? Do you think your measly stupid little vagina could actually hold a baby?

Me: I am having a baby. My baby is growing inside of me. My baby is growing strong.

Subconscious: That affirmation stuff never works.

Me: I am having a baby.

Subconscious: Yah--and you think about chocolate, don't you?

Fibroid Operation

Good thing Chris set the alarm this morning or I might have overslept. My friend Katherine is driving me to the clinic.

When we got to the hospital, Katherine dropped me off at the curb, and wished me well. It all felt so normal, I almost forgot I was on my way to an operation.

Then, the automatic doors to the hospital whooshed open and I went in.

One thing I have to say about this clinic is that the staff is always so on the ball, organized, caring and kind. This morning was no different. As always when I am going to have some type of procedure done here, I feel very taken care of. I was proud of myself for being able to so casually arrive at the hospital alone for the operation. That is what years of dealing with infertility treatments have done to me--I'm braver than I once was, and what would have once been a big deal isn't a big deal anymore.

I prayed a lot as they got me ready for surgery. I pray they don't make any big mistakes during my operation.

For a few moments, I felt utter panic. Alone in that room waiting I missed my husband. I wish he was here.

Then, all the usual stuff happened. I was put on a stretcher and wheeled to an area near the operating room, next to another woman also waiting for surgery. She has been trying to get pregnant for more than a year (I will listen to anyone's story looking for a glimmer of hope). Then it was time.

She and I wished each other well, and it helped to have someone sending me off with good wishes.

I remember little after that. I'm so accustomed now to those last few moments before...wham...lights out.

When I woke up later, I was once again in that horrible recovery room.

Man, I hate this room. It has to be the ugliest, most cheerless, uninteresting recovery room in the world. It looks like it should be in a prison or something (isn't infertility like being in a prison sort of?) Can't they just throw some paint on it? Its like I'm stuck having the same bad dream over and over again.

A nurse asks me how bad my pain is on a scale of 1 to 10 and I always say 10 because I like getting the highest dose of pain medicine possible. The more pain medication, the better.

They say I have to stay 40 minutes, or something like that, before going on to the other waiting room. Every few minutes, I ask if I can go. I can't stand being here. I want to go now. I can't stand waiting here. Now I know how people stuck in nursing homes feel. There is no comfort in this setting. I'm in a lot of pain and I JUST WANT TO GO HOME!

Finally, I am brought to the other waiting room and my husband comes in to see me. Finally, I am allowed to go home. Thank God!

I can't wait to be home and get comfortable in my own bed.

Once in the car, I suddenly feel nauseous.

Everything hurts.

We get on Route 128, and the traffic is thick, slow, unbearable. Why couldn't they let me out before the commuter traffic started? (MOVE THIS BACK)

Cars, cars, cars...rows of cars crammed together.

I start throwing up all over myself.

I don't care. Why so much traffic? I need to throw up again. I open the window and stick my head out. I can barely stand this.

The pain, the car...moving so slow. I want to get home. I need to be home.

My stomach has never hurt this much in my whole life.

This is worse than a caesarean. I can't take this snail-like drive that seems to never end.

Was it not two years ago this month I was on the same road, feeling the same type of sickness, trapped in the same overheated afternoon traffic just like I am now? God help me.

My husband tries to comfort me. "Do you want....?" he asks. No. No! No! I just want to go home. Get me home!

The pain is getting worse. I hate July heat! *Will this ride ever end?.I have no patience for it. I need to be home. They said this would be painful, but this is more than I imagined. Why is it so hot? What is making the traffic go so slow? I need the windows down. No, I need air-conditioning. Put on the air conditioning. Oops, I forgot: we don't have air-conditioning. Please God, kill me right now. Just kill me. No--I take it back. I can't die. I have a daughter. She needs me.*

Forget safety--speed, crash into another car and make the cars move. Stop. I have a daughter. The window looks so good wide open. I am going to jump out. I can't be sentenced to this heat a minute longer. But if I jump, the cars will run over me. ...I can't jump. I am stuck. I am stuck in this heated highway hell forever. I will never escape. God help me. Oh God, please help me. Why is the traffic so bad right now? Why is it so hot? The sun is too bright and too hot. We will never get home. How far to Route 495? How far? Are we almost there? We are starting to go faster. I feel a breeze on my face. I am going to stick my head out the window. I am going to throw my whole ugly fat head out the window. I am going to jump out the window and feel the breeze. No. No. Be patient. When will I feel some relief? I hate the month of July.

Every July is bad for me. It is like the heat magnifies whatever pain I am enduring. God help me. Please God, help me. Be with me. Heal me. Stop this pain. Somebody, please, stop this pain. Chris, drive faster. Get me home. Oh my husband, I love you/Ihate you/this is your fault/it is their fault/it is the doctor's fault/why did they keep me so long and let me get stuck in this?

We are now on Route 495. The Andover exit. *God help me, please, faster, let the exits come faster. The Middleton exit. I am closer. Oh God, it is our exit. We have to drive through a few streets.*

We are almost at my house.

Finally...we pull in the driveway, and I throw open the door and run out, not even stopping to shut the door. I'm home! God, I am home. It feels so good to be home, but the pain doesn't stop. I lie down on the couch.. my beautiful green couch...

My father sits at my feet. He has brought some Young Living Essential Oils to help me. I am dying. Daddy, I am dying. My stomach is on fire. Why am I dying? My daughter is looking at me frightened. I have to be quiet. I need to be quiet. Why can't I shut up? My father starts rubbing my stomach and my feet. It isn't going to help. Nothing is going to help. Chris, call the doctor. Somebody get my doctor. My mother is crying.

My daughter is crying. I am making her scared. I need to stop, be brave, be silent. Oh please...My father keeps rubbing my feet and my stomach.

Could his oils actually be working? I am starting to feel better. He has an oil for stomach pain. He has me drink something. I trust my father. He is smart and kind, and he knows a lot. Please God, let my father help me. Let somebody help me. I am in such pain. My daughter is running around and seems confused. She is scared and I can't help her. Chris, take her upstairs to watch TV. I can't be needed right now. I can't be anything right now. I need to be taken care of. I can't be a good brave mother now. My father keeps rubbing the oils and some of the pain is leaving. Relief. I am actually getting some relief.

I start to feel better. Being so tenderly cared for by my father was a gift I'll never forget. My father has a healing nature, and a true healing ability. I am so grateful he used this on me today. He could have been a doctor, that's how good he is with helping others.
The oils helped stop the terrible pain in my stomach.

My mother tells me that the doctor called while we were driving home to see how I was.

She told my mother everything went well and that she is on the way to vacation, but will talk with me more when she gets back. Thank God— that monster fibroid is gone! Good riddance you terrifying fibroid!

Soon, it is time for my husband to leave for a concert in Boston. Jerk. Complete and utter jerk. I'm sorry to say that, but that is how I feel right now. How could he leave me tonight--for a Monkey's concert? It doesn't matter. I can't flip about this. I have to be cool and just let him think it is fine. His behavior won't matter when I'm 80 years and on my death bed. Then, I want to see at least two children around my bed in those final moments. He probably won't be there anyways and so what he does today won't matter much then. I can't let him be the focus. I can't flip out at him, because he is so sick of this infertility stuff, he'll leave me if I get too difficult, or he'll just stop agreeing to help me have another baby. He deserves some fun. He puts up with a lot. It is fine for him to have fun. Oh God, why is he leaving? I need him. Get a grip. Don't make him suffer for what you want. This is your baby, your project, your obsession, not his. He picked you up and was kind to you on the way home. I have my mother and father here, how much more do I want?

Hopefully he'll remember how nice I was about this.

Plus, we are introducing a friend of ours to a guy tonight. If I have to be without my husband for a night for an old friend to find love, I guess that's okay.

Hey, I can even walk a bit. Everyone said after the fibroid operation I wouldn't be able to walk, but I actually can walk. Now I want to go to bed and sleep. I am so tired.

Day After Fibroid Operation

Today I did not feel half as badly as I expected to feel. First, my husband reported that the friends we were trying to 'fix up' at last night's concert really hit it off.

I thought I wouldn't be able to walk today, but I can walk. Yesterday was harsher than expected, but today I hardly feel any traces of it.

Today, I am going to rest, while my husband takes care of our daughter.

It feels so good to have that fibroid gone. I have an appointment in two weeks for a check-up, and then it is on to the IVF.

Now that the fibroid is gone, I should be able to get pregnant soon.

Thank God!

And A Fibroid Would Have Been So Easy.....

A ton of bricks. Falling on me. Right now.

I went for my first check-up since the fibroid operation.

My doctor very calmly and with no apology whatsoever, told me I did not have a fibroid after all.

Oops.

That explains my amazing recovery. It also explains why I could walk so well after supposedly having a large fibroid removed. It explains why all the pain I was told I was suppose to feel after the operation never came.

And here I was thinking I was some kind of medical marvel.

I'm very confused right now.

The doctor didn't seem upset by her findings.

Or embarrassed.

Or even slightly apologetic.

She told me as if it was no big deal. So I reacted like it was no big deal, because I didn't want to make her feel bad for making such a stupid mistake.

If no fibroid existed, then why am I having so many problems getting pregnant a second time? Now I have no easy answers. The fibroid gave me a way to understand everything.

I am back to square one.

Does this mean I went through all that worry, nausea, and postponement of my IVF for absolutely nothing?

I had thought that changing doctors was a good idea, especially when she discovered a baby-eating fibroid. I thought, 'finally, someone has found the root of all my infertility problems."

As it turns out, she diagnosed me incorrectly.

Now I have to wait until September to do another IVF. Every month that passes means my eggs are one month older.

Having a fibroid made it all so black-and-white.

When I told friends I had a fibroid, many reacted with 'oh yes' 'ah ha' and 'that explains it' and I was told story after story of their sisters, best friends, and co-workers, who had trouble getting pregnant, discovered they had a fibroid, had it removed, and soon had babies born without a hitch. There wasn't something deeply wrong with me on some unexplainable cellular level! It was all the fibroid's fault.

Simple.

Nope. As usual, nothing is that simple.

I have no fibroid. No easy explanation to hang on to. An apology, or an oops, I led you down the wrong path these past few months, would have been nice.

When I thought a fibroid was at the root of all my problems, I sometimes felt slightly carefree. I thought my infertility problems were now going to be simple and straightforward: I have a fibroid. It is killing my babies. It needs to be taken out. Once it is gone, all will be well.

Now I'm left to think that maybe our daughter was a one-in-a-million chance that won't happen again. I feel an almost overwhelming grief.

I want to think this doctor knows what she is doing. She was named by a magazine in our area as one of the best infertility doctors in New England. I like her personality and I trust her.

I just hate that because of this operation my IVF was postponed. I also hate that I had to go through all that pain. For what? For nothing? I told everyone I had a fibroid, even the alternative practitioners I was working with, which might have impacted the treatments they chose to use on me.

And a fibroid would have been so easy...

Preparing for IVF

Lately, everything I do is centered around preparing for the next IVF.

I am stuck in a waiting zone right now. I can't plan ahead for anything, because my plan is to be pregnant, and once I am pregnant, I will quietly nest at home and not do anything else.

Normally, I am an extrovert and I love being with friends. Now I prefer to retreat within myself. I hide more than I ever did before.

Besides, when I come out from my shell, everything feels too real and I am at the mercy of how other people view my chances of becoming pregnant. I can't look at this through anybody's eyes but my own right now. Only in my eyes do I see hope for myself.

God is really the only one I want to talk to about this. He will help me. I believe that. If I didn't believe that, I might just go insane.

I walk around pretending to be part of life's normal routine, when nothing is normal or will be normal until my daughter has a sibling. My husband says I have a one-track mind.

But what else am I suppose to focus on? What is more important than this right now? Not much, at least to me.When I talk out loud about this, I actually feel power leaving my body.

I went up to see Eileen and Dr. Deutsch twice this month. I brought lists of almost every person and memory that might be weighing down my body. It is surprising that old emotional pain, as far back as 1976, can still live in my kidneys, liver, and heart.

Every time I leave their office, I feel joy like I haven't felt in years.

At the same time, one of my best friends and one of the persons I am closest to in this world, Leah, is moving to Portland, Oregan. I could easily be devastated about this, but right now I have to push out all feelings about mostly everything because I have to leave room for this baby to come.

Imagine

I feel so nothing today.

Like I am a bad, flawed person. How could anything good ever happen for me? Nothing I ever do is good. I make so many mistakes. I can't imagine this will ever work out. I'll probably make some big mistake and screw it all up. Other people do this almost without thinking.

I need to stop thinking like this. Today just feels lousy.

Somebody like me doesn't get things. I am not the type...

No, stop. That all changed when my daughter was born. My rotten pattern was permanently altered. I can't think like that anymore.
I am good enough. I deserve a baby.

No I don't. I am a bad person.

Yes, I do.
No I don't.
Shut up!

Transition Time

This must be a time of transitions, of doors opening and closing and I'm not sure what it all means.

I've been at this type of intersection before, where one road closes and an alternative route opens up.

Right now, movement seems to be going on in my life to an extreme. My 98 year old grandmother Maria, who lived on 133 Amesbury St. for the past 29 years, has moved out of her lovely apartment and in with my aunt. The apartment where I slept about a million times and felt so safe in, the one I spent so many happy times visiting, is no longer my grandmother's home.

The white hairbrush on the pretty rose-colored hamper that I always loved to brush my hair with since I was a little girl is not there anymore. How can that be? Shouldn't that brush be in that spot forever?

Suddenly, I can't joke around about 'to grandmother's house we go' since grandma doesn't have a house to go to anymore.

Then, my best friend Leah, who is really more than a best friend, but also a soul mate, a kindred spirit, the kind of friend who sat with you moments after one of the saddest goodbyes of your life, took you by the hands, and somehow made you believe you could survive and go on, is moving to Oregon.

And I start the preparations for my IVF treatments next week.

Beginnings and endings. People leaving, and hopefully, new people arriving.

I've don't like change. One part of me wants to yell at Leah for moving so faraway, "where the hell do you think you are going?"

A part of me wants to say to my grandmother, "Grandma, why did you have to get old? Why can't you stay in your apartment? I miss visiting you. I miss sitting in your kitchen talking to you.

I miss watching TV in the living room with you. I miss showing up at your apartment at 7 a.m. for a cup of coffee. I miss the quiet content times we spent together that that lovely place." Pause. The sobs are coming. Hold on. "Grandma, please don't keep moving away from me like this."

I'm pissed off. Scared. Nostalgic. Teetering on the brink of something.

A part of me wants to run back, hold tight one last time, before life inevitably moves us all on.

Who is coming to replace them? I've found in life that usually when lots of changes occur like this, other things blessedly arrive in their place.

I'm hoping for a little 8 pound somebody.

The Second IVF Begins Now

I am entering a climatic, exciting, and frantic zone.

So much build-up...now reaching a crescendo.

I went this morning for a blood test and I found out that Sunday will be the day of my egg retrieval, Wednesday the implantation, and it all starts tonight with my HCG shot between 7 and 8 p.m.

I've waited since last February for this moment—and it ends up happening on the same weekend as Leah's going away party and my cousin Lori's wedding.

Because the shot needs to be taken by 8 p.m. tonight, I can only stay an hour at Leah's going away party. That is how infertility is--it butts into your life and demands priority regardless of what else is going on.

I built this party up so much to my daughter, talked on and on about "the fun we were going to have at Aunt Leah's party" and now we will basically walk in to the party, say hi, give a few hugs and leave.

I could easily start screaming.

Why is this happening at the same time I have to say goodbye to one the most important people in my life?

A part of me wants to hide out until my baby is born and not deal with anything but baby making. God, I have to get pregnant soon. How many more IVFs will they let me do? How many chances do I get? I can't delve into that murky place right now. This time has got to work.

After all this waiting, it boils down to now. Tonight, finally.

Leah will leave for Portland in a few days. I won't see her after the party tonight. She has been there beside me through everything the past 10 years. How am I going to do without her?

The pain of her leaving is starting to make me physically ache. I can't focus on this or I will fall apart.

I've waited so long for this IVF and now finally it is here. I think I am ready.. I just didn't think it would all start tonight.

We were one of the first ones to arrive at Leah's going away party. I couldn't really explain to her mother why we couldn't stay long. As usual, I feel like I am walking around keeping secrets. Ssh--don't tell anyone. I'm taking my shot tonight. Always, always secrets. Then tomorrow is my cousin's wedding. Chris is stressing about money again because I'm going to see Eileen on Tuesday so she can prepare my body for the implantation Wednesday. Between her and Dr. Deutsch, it will cost about $140. Chris is cranky about this, but I told him I need to go. Good God, to come so far and not do everything possible to make this happen--that would be crazy.

I'm trying not to show Leah how sad I am right now and I'm trying to tell myself that we will always stay close and in touch.
My gut tells me that she will return, but another part of me wonders: will she end up living across the country for the next 20 years? Is one of the most important persons in my life permanently leaving.

I made an attempt to act brave and casual with Leah, talking excitedly about Portland and the wonderful people she is going to meet. I told her how proud I was of her for making this daring move.

I am just feeling very sad for myself.

Around 6:45 p.m., we say goodbye. I feel selfish leaving the party so early, but the shot has to be priority right now. Leah and I stood at the door of the old Grange hall, hugging tightly. Leah starts to cry, and I am just about overwhelmed by a tidal wave of grief. I try to hold it back. I can't let myself despair over her departure. She is doing what she needs to do to create the life she wants, and I am doing what I need to do to create the life I want.

Oh, if only it was all so cut and dry. My dear beloved, best friend Leah is leaving!

We got home, and at exactly 8 o'clock, Chris gave me the shot. Now, my ovaries are cooking with eggs. Oh God, please let me get pregnant. Please God, make this work. I've done so much, prepared and waited so long, please God don't let me be disappointed.

Cousin Lori's Wedding and the IVF

Today was my cousin Lori's wedding. It was absolutely beautiful and I was thrilled to be there. Amber looked so pretty in her dress. Bringing her to the wedding meant so much to me. Everything takes on a different hue when I'm with her. She loved the cake. She loved the outdoor wedding. She loved Lori's dress. She loved seeing Lori dance with her husband Bob. She loved dancing and twirling with me and Chris, and really, there is nothing I love better than dancing and twirling with my little girl.

Despite all this happiness, I felt like I was walking around with a big ticking time-bomb of a secret, as if people looked at me closely enough, they could see that I am a walking mound of infertility drugs.

I didn't eat a piece of wedding cake because I want to make sure my body is in optimum condition for the retrievel tomorrow.

There is a eerie stress level that accompanies an IVF. It is so completely unnatural in one way, and yet so natural in another way to be doing whatever is needed to expand our family. I wonder what it must be like for people who can simply make love and then discover—surprise!-- they are pregnant. Something that happens so naturally for millions of people is a faraway reality for me.

Today, surrounded by the normalcy of a man and woman getting married, I felt like a big fake because there is nothing even near normal in my reality right now. Doing an IVF is like walking into a steel metal futuristic world, where all the old comforts are gone and in their place are new technologies that in order to work cannot allow in even a trace of the old softness. Imagine the comfort, safety, and casual joys of quilts, puppies, old-fashioned porches and children playing outside on a spring day. Then imagine the opposite of all that. That is what an IVF is like.

While dancing with my daughter, I thought: Am I the first person in my family who ever got a baby this way?

I looked around at all my cousins and their babies and their babies' babies, and my aunts and my grandmother and my mother, and I thought: all these women had babies the good, old-fashioned way, and me, always so odd, had my baby come to life through heavy infertility medications and weird scientific procedures.

And you know what? I didn't care. As I danced with my beautiful daughter, I thought, 'she is here, and if my road was different to get her here, so be it.' Thank God I was born now, and not 100 years ago.

As strange, weird and oddball as I am, I was not a childless woman at this wedding today, but like all my aunts and cousins and their babies and their babies' babies and my aunts and my grandmother and my mother, I am a mother now too.

Regardless of how I am making a family, I am making one. Ultimately, that is what matters most.

9/11

The day started out sunny. A bright, beautiful sunny. The kind of sunny that gives you a wink and a nod that it is going to be a great day.

I am driving down Route 95 heading to Portland, Maine to see Eileen and Dr. Deutsch. I am in high spirits.

Two days ago, they retrieved ten eggs from me. Ten! Tomorrow they will implant them. With God's help, I could be pregnant soon.

I am thankful as I drive that today the weather is beautiful. So beautiful. Alone, on a highway that is a joy to drive, the radio on as my companion, I listen to the morning DJs do hilariously awlful pranks on unsuspecting listeners.

I am feeling good.

Then, a disc jockey says he can't believe that he just saw on TV a plane crash into the World Trade Center in New York.

I think: are they replaying some old news clip from long ago? I never heard about this. I don't always follow the news as closely as I should....

The disc jockey sounds upset. He says he can't believe that now a second plane is crashing into another tower. Is this some kind of sick joke? I switch the station in disgust. What a rotten disc jockey. It is one thing to phone some unsuspecting listener and tell them you are calling from the dog pound, or a local auto dealer, or the courthouse, and tease them into thinking they are being fined or something. It is another thing to play a horrible joke about planes crashing into buildings.

As much as I love a good joke, this went too far.

But as I switch from station to station, I keep hearing more and more of the same thing. Two planes, two towers, New York City.

What is going on?

I don't want to listen anymore. This cannot be happening. I switch the channels on the radio faster and faster.

I no longer see the sunshine or the highway or anything else. The sun is still there, the day is still beautiful, but I can't see it, feel it, anymore.

By now, I know something wicked has happened. Something unimaginable. People on the radio are crying. Screaming. Confused. Even the disc jockeys and news people seem to be falling apart. Not today. Oh God, not today, not any day.

I finally arrive for my 10 o'clock appointment with Eileen. A few people are crying and people are going to an office upstairs to watch TV.

Eileen looks upset. We go into the room where she does her treatments. But today, she is not herself. Her brother lives in New York City and she can't get through to him. She doesn't know how he is. She starts my treatment, lowers her head and begins to sob.

She prays out loud, asking God to please help those people suffering in those towers, people that could be dying or burning to death. She says there must be a reason I am there with her at this time. I don't say anything. I feel so confused.

Never in my life have I felt so torn between my own needs and the pressing needs of the larger world around me. Tomorrow is the IVF I have waited for the past eight months. It is the IVF I am counting on to give me a baby and give my daughter a sibling. It is the IVF that I haven't stopped thinking about since last February. It is the IVF I have spent thousands of dollars preparing for. It is the IVF that has given me hope when all I felt was despair and rage.

I need Eileen to do a good job right now. I know I am selfish for thinking that. Then it hits me what is really happening to good wonderful people in those towers and I can't stay hidden from the truth anymore. The sadness hits me so hard. If I let my feelings descend any further, I am heading fast towards the brink of hysterical.

Eileen is not going to be able to focus. I know that. Her treatment was suppose to prepare my body to receive. I am trying to tell myself I can get pregnant whether this session with Eileen goes well or not. I tell myself this, but I know the timing of this cannot be worse for me.

Can I pretend this is not happening? Can I pretend that my country is safe and people in New York are going about their business as usual? Is it right to try and shut this out to save myself and my potential unborn babies? Or do I join everyone else and go insane? Do I hold tight to my sanity as a way to hold on to my chance of getting pregnant?

Eileen cannot continue. I am disappointed, but I understand. Dr. Deutsch comes in and does his treatment.

Driving home, I listen to the radio.

Oh my God, all my thoughts about tomorrow's IVF leave and I begin to cry. This is too horrible! I start screaming, sobbing, crying. Loudly, profusely. Getting ready for the IVF these past few weeks has made me feel very weary, but now everything feels unbearably sad like never before.

I get home and my husband is watching on TV a replay of what happened. Our daughter begins to cry. Does she understand what is happening?

I begin to watch the nightmare too...but it is too horrible. I cannot fall into the misery of this event. This is not happening, I tell my husband, it is not happening. It has never happened. I will lie to my body. I will trick my body and not let it know what unspeakableness has occurred today.

I cannot do this/I have to save myself/ My body will not get pregnant if it is laden down with sadness.

I ask my husband to shut off the TV. At first, he protests. He is sad, confused, needing to watch. I beg him, explaining that I can't take all the sadness. I can't take the whole IVF thing during an attack on my country. I wonder if we should even do the IVF tomorrow.

Will the hospital be blown up next? Is it safe to go to a public place tomorrow? Will there be a terrorist attack somewhere on the highway as we are driving?

There is no way I will can pregnant with the level of despair I am feeling. This is so crazy and unfair.

Just as it has been for months, I am completely alone in what I have to do--banished to some remote island where my reality has to be completely different than everyone elses. At a time when I have every right to wail and scream and cry, I'm not allowed. I have to stay disciplined, on track, focused.

Damn, this is too much.

Now the crazy, lonely, forbidden, desolate world I've inhabited in my head for the past few months is spreading out everywhere around me. I'm not the only one mourning, and it makes my pain more intense.

It is like everything in my head is playing itself out in some dark national nightmare.

This is not happening. This is not happening. If I keep telling myself this is not happening, maybe it will go away. Please God, make this not be real.

Tonight, I lay in bed praying. Please God, help the firefighters, the people in the towers, the people on those planes, everyone. I am in a tug-of-war: sad for the suffering of people I haven't met, sad for my babies that I haven't met, sad for myself, and hysterical for the people who have lost their lives and for their families.

It is all too much.

The world feels heavy tonight. Sad, heavy, and upside down.

I am trying to retreat into my own head, just as I have done for the past several months, but I can't. The reality of this is beyond what I can bear.

I must sneak away to my own inside place or I'll never get pregnant and my daughter will end up without a brother or sister.

How can this be happening? How? To me! To the country where I live! To those innocent people in the World Trade Center! How? Why now?

I want to shut my eyes and block my ears. I am being robbed of my future babies. If I let them, my baby will be another casualty in this tragedy. Those terrorists are not going to steal my baby who I am suppose to conceive tomorrow. I won't let them take this one...I will get pregnant tomorrow!

I am suppose to have the transfer tomorrow, but the clinic doesn't guarantee it until the morning when they know for sure the embryos survived the transfer. Maybe all my embroys will die and I'll end up with no IVF tomorrow. I don't think I could take that right now.

God help us all tonight.

9/12 Day of IVF

Today, the day I have waited for since last February has finally arrived. The day I planned for, drept about, prayed day and night about, has finally arrived. Could I have ever imagined worse timing?

We got up and waited for the call from the nurse. I am getting panicky that maybe all my embryos have died.

Finally, we get the call that I have three viable embryos. Seven died. Man, all the things I did and still seven died.

My eggs aren't good quality. Will my three embryos die in a day or two also?

For a moment, I want to cancel the IVF.

Everything felt surreal on the drive to the clinic. I looked at the cars around me and wondered, are you the car carrying a bomb? I pray for safety. I pray for help. I don't know where to put my mind.

At the hospital, we head to the IVF floor.

The whole world feels upside down, and I think: how upside down is my world that my IVF falls on the day after one of the most horrific and heartbreaking national disasters of all time?

Everyone is acting differently today. The nurses are putting on a good face, trying to pretend that everything is normal, but nothing is normal.

I can't help but think: is this hospital the next target?

They tell me my eggs are showing lots of damage and they are a C quality. Great. Two eggs are rated poor quality and one fair. I wish they didn't tell me this. How in the world can I make a baby with such poor egg quality?

Dr. M does the transfer. She is positive, gentle, and says nice things.

I try to be positive, but all I can think of is the poor quality of my eggs. I wish I didn't know that most of my eggs are considered a C or D. This is too weird, too science fictiony. I just want a baby, but knowing every little thing like egg quality, makes it all seem eerie, dark and impossible.

This time, after the transfer, I lay as long as I am suppose to. I drank less water than last time, so holding my pee isn't as bad.

We don't talk much on the way home. The world feels so heavy right now

Tonight's Explosion

It all came to a head tonight. An explosion of sorts. A dam-ready to burst.

It is the day after my transfer, and my husband decides he will go into work at 3 o'clock in the morning so he can come home early tomorrow to watch our daughter and give me a chance to a rest.

His job sometimes allows him to make his own schedule.

He reasons that while me and my daughter are sleeping, he might as well work. The idea being, the more rest I have, the better chance I have of getting pregnant.

The plan seems good. Only somewhere around 3:30 p.m. my daughter wakes up crying. I rock her to sleep, but then I am left wide awake in the middle of a dark lonely night.

Such a dark lonely night.

The veil is lifted and it is all there. The World Trade Center, terrorism, planes flying into buildings, people dying, New York City under attack, my IVF.

I feel crazy, looney, thrust into some type of big screen terror flick, dozens of horrifying images playing out in my head. This seems like a bad movie gone wrong. I start to cry, a heavy, throbbing thundering cry.

It is a cry I have cried before on my darkest of days, and I never forget when I cry this way. I fall to my knees and cry louder. I don't care that I have woken up my daughter. I don't care that she is crying now. I don't care, because my own sobs keep coming louder and louder and I can't stop. I am on my knees now, screaming for help, because the World Trade Center was attacked and the IVF I have waited so long for landed on the same week I can't stop crying. I cry and cry, and for a moment, I see myself in a snapshot of darkness and it becomes a permanent part of my memory, in the same way that those other times I have cried like this before have become.

I call my husband at work. Please come home, I beg. He is annoyed. He is tired of all my neediness. It is too much for him. He is ready to quit. He wonders why we are putting ourselves through this. He doesn't seem to care whether I get pregnant or not. He feels like he already did enough. Now, I am crying for more? I need him to come home. I need him to care for our daughter. I can't deal with her crying right now.
He reluctantly agrees to come home. He hates me, but I don't care. I just need him here. I don't care that he will have to go back to work later.

I don't care about anything. I turn on the home and garden channel. My daughter calms down.

I hold her and try to pretend that the world is still as pretty as all those lovely homes on TV. I am scared and alone, and if the world falls apart tonight, I want my husband home with me, even if he hates me for it.

Red Alert

It has been a long, drawn-out, painstakingly agonizing ten days since my IVF. Pretty much, all I think about, except for my daughter, is that I have to be pregnant this time.

My mind runs in circles: Am I pregnant? I am pregnant! Yes, I know I am pregnant. I am so happy ! I did it! No, I'm not pregnant. I am destroyed, depressed, a loser. I am not pregnant/ I have to be pregnant/I am not pregnant/I am/Am not/Am.

Am I pregnant? Yes, I am pregnant. My baby is on the way. My mood soars. No, it isn't going to happen. I am defeated, murdered, withered and grasping for breath. Please God."

On and on it goes.

There are moments of relief, of course, like when I look at my daughter's most beautiful face and I thank God for her existence. But the more I fall in love with her, the more frantic I become to get her a brother or sister.

Today, I hit an extreme low. All day, I feel sad and weird.

Dr. Zhu gave me an herbal drink to help me get pregnant that I am suppose to take only once every few days. But today, I can't follow his instructions. Every few minutes, I go to the refrigerator and take a slug out of the bottle. I'm not suppose to do this, but I can't stop. I have to do something to make me get pregnant! I am drunk on Chinese herbs!

I also start slugging down liquid iron. I know I am not even suppose to take this, but I can't seem to stop.

I have to do something, take something...now I take a red raspberry herb. I took these when I was trying to get pregnant with my daughter...maybe they will help now.

Then I take two more vitamins. Then I drink more of Dr. Zhu's herbs.

"You're not suppose to be doing that," my husband says. Ouch—I'm caught!

I try to convince him I know what I'm doing.

He says cut it out.

What a jerk.

I need to get away from him. I go outside to sit on the front steps and pray.

It is an incredibly beautiful sunny autumn day. In a few hours, we are going to a party at my cousin's house. I am not in the mood for a party. I am overcome by some new mutant breed of desperateness.

Being outside in the sunshine makes me feel a little better. Then my husband says it is time to get ready for the party. He is always bugging me. Good lord, just leave me alone.

He goes back in the house and I keep praying. The sun is beautiful and I feel close to God right now. I also feel a raw desperateness I hate feeling that won't let up for a moment and give me a break.

I feel overwhelmingly sad right now and I don't know why.

A few minutes later, I head into the bathroom to start getting ready for the party and I see exactly why I felt so desperate: blood.

No God, not after all this! No! Please God, no blood.

No Blood! I scream for my husband.

When I tell him the blood has come, he looks so sad. I try tell myself that a woman can get her period and still be pregnant.

I phone the clinic's emergency hotline to ask them what they think I should do. A nurse calls back. I tell her I did an IVF and now I am bleeding

I ask her if I could still be pregnant despite the blood.

She is aggravated and instructs me to just come in for my pregnancy test in a few days. I start asking questions: could I still be pregnant? Is there any hope?

The nurse says little, yah, I could be pregnant. No, she can't tell me what chance there is. She seems angry. I don't care. I need answers.

At my cousin's party, I am quiet. I tell everyone I don't feel well. I sit in the kids playroom and watch my daughter play. I want to say: guess what everybody? I did an IVF two weeks ago and today I got my period. Chances are I blew this like I blow most things in my life.

No one could possibility understand how alone I feel right now, how this could mean that my dream of creating a happy family life for my child is disappearing.

Maybe I shouldn't have drank so many herbs.
I can't think about that...can't deal with it being my fault. My husband wants to go down this road, but I won't let him. He has no idea how helpless I felt today, and compelled I was to drink and take things, and pray and take and drink again.

I don't even try to hide my glumness at the party. I sit, slumped in a big comfy old-fashioned recliner, watching my daughter play with other children. Thank God they have this playroom for the kids, or I would have been forced to socialize the whole night.

The pain inside me is so intense that hiding it is impossible. Tonight I have absolutely nothing to say to anybody. I can only look at my beloved daughter and watch her play. Through her, I speak. Through her, I live.

Through her, I glimpse a little of life's happiness. For myself, there is absolutely nothing left to say tonight.

I go to the clinic on Tuesday. I am clinging to the small slight hope that maybe I am still pregnant.

The blood is flowing and flowing. My red alert desperation tracking device worked loud and clear.

I guess when you've lost many, many times before, you get pretty good at knowing when you are about to lose again.

Worst News

Today was my pregnancy test. I think I know the answer.

The nurse's called later that day: No, I'm not pregnant. I did, however, have a chemical pregnancy however and it did not continue. The words shake me to the core. What is this thing called chemical pregnancy?

Tell me everything, explain this to me, I ask. Why did this happen? Was it my eggs? Is it because of the quality of my eggs?

I am not trying to be a pain, but I need answers.

The nurse is annoyed. She barely answers my questions.

No, I am not crazy. I just want an explanation.

The nurse is cold, aloof, off-putting. As if I have no right to ask so many questions.

I dial the clinic again and get the voice mail for my nursing team. I leave a question.

A few minutes later, I call again. I leave another question. I call again 12 minutes later. I have more questions. I can't stop calling. I can't stop asking questions. I need answers. No one is giving me answers. No one is explaining why this happened. I dial again, and leave more questions.

I need to know. Am I on the wrong medication?

What is going on with me? I need information. If only I could understand this. Why isn't anyone telling me anything?

One nurse in particular is extremely rude to me. She acts as if I'm complaining about an order gone wrong at a drive through. She doesn't have time for me and I know she thinks I'm crazy. Maybe I am crazy. Yes, I am crazy today. Who can blame me? Who can blame me for being crazy? What am I suppose to be--rational after all this?

I dial again and leave more questions. I can't stop even though I know I should. No one is answering me! No one is helping me! I feel compelled to act. Give me answers! Give me information! Please, tell me right now what went wrong and why.

Finally, a kind nurse calls me back. Her name is Chris and she is very sympathetic. She tries to answer my questions, but she doesn't have the answers.

I ask her if she thinks I'll ever get pregnant again. She tries to sound hopeful, without giving me false hope that could make the clinic liable. I appreciate her kindness and trying to answer my questions the best she could. She is so different from the other nurses.

I will never forget the kindness of this nurse who called me back.

I have so many questions. I need to make an appointment with my doctor to discuss everything about my treatment, from the amount of progesterone I am given, to my medication. Something is wrong.
I can't believe this is happening!
I feel a crazy inconsolable kind of anger and helplessness.

A few minutes later, a counselor from the clinic calls to see how I am doing. Probably that mean nurse reported me, told the counselor to call the crazy woman leaving too many messages on the voice mail. I quickly get a grip and feign saneness while I talk to her. I'm frightened she will report that I am too nuts to go through another IVF.

I hate this counselor. She has to be the most insensitive, cruel counselor imaginable. She tells me some awful statistic on women my age getting pregnant. She goes on to list all the problems that can be expected at my age. Is that what she thinks is going to comfort me? What a freakin' idiot! I wish I could report her to someone, but if I do, she will label me as psychotic and they will kick me out of the clinic.

Someday I'll write a letter to the clinic telling them about the complete insensitivity of this supposed counselor.

I wonder how many other woman she made feel hopeless during their darkest moments. She has no right to hold this position, but I need to stay quiet right now and pretend I am okay.

I tell her I feel fine. Yes, I am disappointed, I say casually, but I'll get over it. She seems to accept that. The idiot can be tricked so easily. I thank her for calling. She asks if I want an appointment, and instead of saying no, I tell her I have my daughter to care for and getting a sitter is hard, but yes, eventually I would love to come in for an appointment.

What a stupid lady. She falls for it, hook, line and sinker. I hate playing this game with her, but she scares me.

She is mean enough and lacks insight in such full measure that if I tick her off in any way, she will say I'm not psychologically fit to handle another IVF. So I pull myself together during this phone call and I act like I'm fine and okay about this pregnancy gone wrong, not a woman with any emotion, thank you.

My husband seems confused too. Has the possibility of having another baby already escaped us? I go crazy at the thought.
I have a million questions and no answers. This was not at all what I expected.

Chemical Pregnancy Nightmare

Why didn't I get pregnant this time?

No one seems to be able to tell me why.

I have an appointment to talk with my doctor. I mailed her a letter with 20 questions, so that she can take some time and review my particular case before we meet.

Am I on the right medicine?

Am I getting enough progesterone?

Do I need some type of test to determine whether there is a virus in my body causing these problems?
And if so, do I need a strong and swift antibiotic to be rid of this infection?

I hope sending the questions ahead of time will make it possible for her to thoroughly research all my questions.

I want everyone to just go away and leave me alone.

Devastating Meeting

Today was my meeting with Dr. N. I woke up excited. Finally! I'll get some answers! She has my questions and had lots of time to research them.

I have been reading about some new medications, and there are some medicines out there that seem to suit me. I am requesting a change.

I wore my red suit, with the idea that maybe, if I looked professional, she would take me seriously. Boy, was I in for a surprise.

Instead of going over the questions, she immediately began talking about the number of messages I left on the nursing team's voice mail. She alluded to the fact that her nurses were aggravated with me.

Immediately, I knew this meeting wasn't going in a good direction.

I'm being tested right now, I thought, and I better remain cool if I ever want the chance to do another IVF at this clinic again.

I immediately apologized for my persistent phone calls, and explained that a first, I was very upset.

Then she asked if I was okay now, and if I felt I was able to take doing another IVF.

"I'm fine," I smiled convincingly "I was upset, but I'm over it. I understand these things happen."

Hah! I really wanted to say: Doctor, I'm still a basket case, but obviously, you, like everyone else around here, wants me to feel no emotion at all.

You prefer me to be just another quiet little number in the pecking order. Take my disappointment and shove it down. Ask no questions. Make no demands. Make no waves. Exactly what everyone wants out of women everywhere--to stay silent and just be good little soldiers who do as they are told without ever protesting or questioning or feeling.

That's right ladies, you should feel nothing regardless of what you are going through. Say nothing, accept whatever is handed to you without any emotion at all. And you, being a women doctor, should know better, teach your nurses better, understand more. I expected more from you, but you are no different than the people who have wanted to silence women for years. I get it.

I'm too much work, too much hassle, and you have no time to answer 22 questions. I understand the rules here: passion, sadness, hysteria, desperation, is in no way allowed. I understand. I am suppose to do this without feeling.

I'm suppose to take the bad news and cry silently alone, and never bother anyone with my pain.

Then she went on to suggest that maybe I take some test to determine my ovarian reserve and chances of getting pregnant. No way, I think, I am not taking some test so you can label me unable to conceive and then insurance will stop all my treatment.

I tell her maybe later, it sounds good, but I want to do another IVF first.

She looks at me quite seriously and tells me that because of the amount of medication I need, it looks as if my eggs are at the bottom of the barrel.

Everything stops for a minute. The little trickle of hope I had left oozes away. I didn't expect this.

She says for my age, I need way too much medication. She questions if I ever smoked, and I tell her I never even tried a cigarette in my life. She seems to not believe me, and asks again. I repeat that I've never even tried a cigarette in my life.

She now recommends that I look into donor eggs, and I think: no, I'm not doing that.

Then I tell her that despite all my problems, I think I still have a chance of having one more child. "All I need is for one egg to turn out right," I say, trying to sound reasonable, logical, defending myself against her attack, but most of all fighting the hopelessness building inside me.

"Maybe," she says, with an expression that means "keep dreaming dummy."I ask her if she wants to go over any of my questions. She glances quickly at them. It is obvious she hasn't gone over them. She says they don't apply.

I ask about changing my medication. She doesn't want to consider it right now.

I rise to leave. We shake hands and I pretend I am okay.

I thank her for her time.

Once I get in the car, I feel wildly, frantically angry. I am stunned. I can't even cry. I drive home in a daze. Her words ring in my head: your eggs are the bottom of the barrel. Your eggs are bottom of the barrel...your eggs are bottom of the barrel."

I never realized it was this bad. Regardless of everything I've gone through, I never felt like my time was up.

My time can't be up! I need another baby--I need a baby for my daughter! I can't accept this...I can't live with this.

I start to pray. I pray and I pray and I pray, because I know under no uncertain terms that it will only be through God's help that I will ever get a baby now.

I am at such a desperate point. Her words have nearly broken my will and spirit. Thank God I know God. Thank God I can pray to God. If I didn't have God and His gift of prayer, I would give up right now.

After I pray, for some reason I can't explain, I stop on the way home at a big alternative supermarket in my area and go directly to their book section.

I am searching for hope.

I start reading a book on women's health written by Christine Northrup, *Women's Bodies, Women's Wisdom* and I come upon her chapter on reproduction and fertility.

She writes that in other cultures, it is perfectly normal for women in their late 40s to have babies. She thinks that some of the infertility problems in the United States are because women are told they are too old to have babies in their 30s. This is wrong, she says, and the problems stem primarily from lifestyle, eating habits and stress.

A little bit of hope returns, and I thank God for physicians like Dr, Northrup who give women hope, instead of ripping it away like Dr. M.

I had switched to Dr. M I assumed that because she was a woman, she would have more empathy and more of a bedside manner than Dr. S., but I was wrong.

First, she misdiagnosed me with a fibroid and now she calls my eggs bottom of the barrel.

She obviously doesn't like to be hassled or bothered, and someone like me, who asked too much of her nursing team and mailed her 22 questions, was obviously too much work.

When I got home, a neighbor who had undergone infertility treatments was visiting. She recommended I switch to her doctor, who was in the same clinic.

I went upstairs to call my mother. I desperately needed to talk to my mother. It is times like these that it is my mother's voice I need to hear above all others.

There are few people on this earth who you can always count on to provide you with hope, but I am fortunate enough to say regardless of whatever has happened in my life, my mother has always given me hope.
My brilliant mother always understands that bottom line: hope will get a person through. If she didn't do this, I don't know if I would have ever gotten past some of the disappointments in my life.

My mother is also very intelligent. She gave me this brilliant advice, "That doctor doesn't believe you can have a baby. I know you can. Change doctors. Do it today, immediately. If she is telling you this stuff, go to another doctor who is willing to work with you."

My mother was right. Why was I giving her opinion of my fertility so much power? My mother is right—let me see what another doctor has to say. I hung up with my mother, and immediately phoned the clinic to have my records transferred to Dr. G, my neighbor's doctor.

I set up an appointment for next week and mailed him the same 22 questions I had given Dr. M.

Dr. M has no idea what she did to me. If not for God and my mother, I might just give up on ever having another biological child. What kind of monster is she? Who is this doctor that thinks it is okay to rip a person's heart out? Maybe in her mind, she really thinks there is no hope for me.

Maybe she thinks I'm so crazy, that it is better to remove all hope from me.

Well, maybe I am a bit crazy, but I'm not so crazy as to stop trying.

She took some of the fight out of me today. I went there looking for answers and instead I got put in my place. A demanding, out-of-control, strong-willed woman being put in her place, ironically, by another woman. Not at all what I expected when I chose this doctor.

Tonight, in bed, anger and rage came over me. I wanted to phone the clinic and leave 100 nasty messages about this doctor and her cowardly nursing team.

My husband stopped me.

"Give me the phone," I cried. "They all deserve to be told off! She deserves me to tell her what I think of her!"

"No, don't blow it," he warned.

"I don't want to ever go back to that clinic. I want to go to another clinic. She deserves to be told off," I say.

"Don't do it. If you do, you can't go back there. Just do another IVF and see what happens," he says reasonably.

"I can't stand it. I have to tell her off," I cry.

"Paula, don't blow this. If you tell them off, they will think you are crazy and they won't let you do another IVF. Not there, and maybe nowhere else either. Just do the IVF and maybe you'll get a baby next time," he says this with such reassurance that I calm down.

"You are right," I said. "But when I have my next baby, I am going to march into her office and say, "SEE YOU JERK! SEE THIS BEAUTIFUL BABY! THIS IS WHAT BOTTOM OF THE BARREL LOOKS LIKE!!!"

Jealous and Ashamed Of It

I am turning more and more inward, Being with people, particularly certain people, is getting harder and harder.

Tonight was a case in point.

A friend of ours got married last year to a wonderful girl, and now They are moving back to her hometown next week. We invited them over for a farewell dinner.

A few days ago, we also found out she is pregnant.

Tonight, I could hardly stand the way they joked about the surprise of it all. Surprise? What is it like to get a baby as a surprise? No work, no heart break...just SURPRISE!

Every jealous bone in my body came popping out.

Right now, I can hardly stand knowing that some people just make love and get pregnant. Of course, I know that happens all the time, but to have someone in my house, joking about getting pregnant, not understanding that in my world, pregnancy is accompanied by lots and lots of shots, lots and lots of blood tests, lots and lots of calls from nurses, and lots and lots of nos, is hard.

My friend's wife comes from a family of eight kids. She is 28 years old. They've been married barely over a year.

When I hesitated to let her have chocolate, remembering that chocolate is not recommended for high risk pregnancies, she ate it anyways without a care in the world. What is that like? Having babies is going to be no big deal for her. She said she definitely wants at least one more baby. And she said it in a way that you know she could have whatever number of children she wanted. One more, three more, six more..she will have the choice in creating whatever size family she wants. What is that like?

It was hard hearing about how they are going to living right next door to some of her siblings, who also have lots of kids. Great...lots of ready-made friends and cousins for her baby!

It was also hard hearing how excited her sisters are for her, while I am feeling so alone right now, my daughter without cousins and without a sibling.

Finally, I couldn't stand it anymore. All I kept thinking was: I should be pregnant. Not her. What did she do to earn this pregnancy? What suffering has she done?

I know this is a terrible way to think, but I couldn't shake the feeling of how unfair it is that some people can get pregnant without hardly even trying.

I told everyone that I was sick and took my daughter and went up to bed.

When I got to the top of the stairs, I felt such relief. Ah, escape!

Right now, the only place in this world I feel safe is in my bedroom, alone, faraway from reality.

After they left. I told my husband I wished he never invited them over.

He didn't understand and scolded me for being a lousy friend.

I am not in the mood for his lectures.

Ever since that stupid Dr. M. decided to crack my will in half, I am sad beyond words.

I am only happy when I'm with my daughter, but there is a constant ache inside me that maybe no more children may be coming to me. How dare Dr. M steal my hope away. What now? What next?

I felt so trapped in my own house tonight--trapped with two people that in any other circumstance I would love spending time with--but in the world I'm inhabiting right now, when all that matters is getting pregnant, I couldn't stand being with them.

I was jealous of her nausea and had no stomach for her stories about morning sickness.

Give me the nausea. Give me the morning sickness. Give me the baby. Give me the opportunity to choose the number of siblings my daughter has.

All I want to do right now is be alone with my daughter and feel sorry for myself.

Fair Time

A darkness has come over me I am trying to conjure up the optimism and hope I had last spring, when I was in full throttle healing mode, but I can't.

It isn't that easy to get revved up again. Where did all that healing get me? No pregnancy and a bad diagnosis from my doctor?

What if I took that awlful test she recommended and the results were that my chances of ever getting pregnant were zero? What do I do then?

If I think too long, a scream builds in my throat. How wrong it would be if my biological clock is up.

I don't want to talk about this with anyone. It seems that beneath the smiles and nods, people mostly agree with my doctor.
My husband joins me in the world of miracles and prayer. He is ready to believe despite the physical evidence around us, and right now, except for my parents, he is the only one I can trust with this.

I understand that I am extremely fortunate to have my daughter, but it is because of my love s for her that I desperately want to give her a sibling. Am I asking too much?

Is it so wrong of me to want for her what millions and billions of other children around the world have? A sibling to grow up with, a lifelong friend, someone to share her childhood with?

I am not giving up just because my doctor says I should. My daughter deserves better from me than that.

Today was a big fair in our area. We planned to take our daughter and meet up with some friends. My heart was barely in it. While I was excited for my daughter to try fried dough and see elephants and ponies, it hurts to be with lots of people right now.

I don't know why, but it seems everyone we ran into at the fair was there with their adult brothers and sisters.

We ran into one friend who was there with her younger brother. When her brother walked away, she whispered about the surprise anniversary party she was throwing him and his wife. Normally, this wouldn't bother me, but today, anything related to siblings hurt a lot.

Then I ran into a friend who is pregnant with twins, already has two children, and four siblings of her own. How lucky can one person get? I am jealous. What is it like to be surrounded by family and able to give this gift to the next generation?

Then some of my husband's cousins met up with us. Of course, they arrive two brothers with their sister. Fairs must bring out some sort of family togetherness thing or something. I can't wait to go home and hide in my bedroom. But when we get home, a bunch of our friends from the fair come over too.

Our friend who lives in our basement complains that it is too hot in the house, and I say that I am cold. Then (he definitely picked the wrong day to say this) he says, "ah, the sister I never wanted."

Wow—bad timing. I took my daughter and marched up to my bedroom.

Being referred to as an unwanted sister was not exactly what I needed to hear today.

I can't let my daughter down. She deserves to have the safety of a brother or sister that all those people I saw today have.

God help me, what if my time is up? What if my eggs are mostly gone and the ones left are so damaged that no baby can ever come from them? What then....?

I pray and I pray and I pray, because prayer is all I have left.

Phone Conference With New Doctor

Today was my first meeting with my new doctor. I didn't feel well, so I phoned the clinic to see if our first conference could be on the telephone. Surprisingly, the doctor agreed without a hitch.

I immediately felt better when I heard the doctor's voice. He was kind. He wasn't rushed and he had answers to almost all of my 22 questions. He agreed that it was time to change medications, and had already been thinking of the medication I requested.

Let me say it again: he was already considering the new medication I was requesting What a good sign! We were on the same page. So different from Dr. M who wouldn't even consider trying a new medication on me!

Then, as we talked, he said,"considering everything, I see no reason why you can't have another baby."

Hallelujah!

Give that doctor a gold star, a medal, some type of award!

His words gave me hope!

Now that is what a doctor is suppose to do!

We agreed I would phone his nurses on Day One of my next period. Thank God, and my mother, that I changed doctors. What a difference!

If I had stayed with that other doctor, she would never have changed my medication, and because she saw no hope for me, she would not have done anything to help me.

In contrast, this doctor was open and willing to try something new.

Was didn't Dr. M. consider changing my medicine? Did a patient like me, who wanted to try again and again, threaten to screw up the statistics that made her the most successful infertility doctor in New England?

My new doctor sees hope for me! I hate caring so much what authority figures think, but considering he is on my side, I am pretty excited.

Could this make the difference? I hope so.

Riding the See-Saw

A few days ago, I got an e-mail from a friend who said pregnancy at 34 was difficult for her, and that made me slightly depressed all day.

A friend in my department at work just announced she is pregnant. She is 42+ and I am elated--there is hope for me too!

My moods go up and down all day just like that, based on information I receive on pregnancy.

A friend confides that his girlfriend is 42 and doctors predicted they couldn't have children. But she had a baby boy last month! Score another for hope!

Up and down, up and down. It is hard to be constantly riding the see-saw of hope and despair.

We took my daughter to the park today and it was beautiful. The air warm. The leaves a color feast.

Sometimes at the park I feel lonely. So many people come and go, and we say hi to them all, but chances are we'll never see them again.

I sometimes wish I could make friends with all of them, that somehow more people would come into my life. I feel sad when I see my daughter so much wanting to connect with children who are either too shy or already have a set of friends/cousins/siblings/whatever to meet their social/emotional needs.

It is hard to talk about this with most people. When people say things like, 'if God wants you to have another baby, you will." My question is: what if God doesn't want me to have another baby? What then?"

Then I want to say: "Why would God dislike me so much that He wouldn't want me to have another baby?'

A part of me wants to say, "Shut up! Of course God wants my daughter to have a sibling. Cut the crap." No one would ever dare tell a cancer victim fighting for their life, "If God wants you to live, you will."
But in the world of infertility, people still feel they have some right to make you feel like maybe God isn't in with you on your plans.

A Ride to Maine with Leah

Leah and I both had appointments with Dr. Deutsch today, and so we drove up to Maine together. She moved back from Portland—thank God!

On the way up, Leah asked me how do I know I will get pregnant again. She asked in a positive let's-have-some-heartfelt-talk kind of way.

Usually, I love when she asks me these kind of questions. Normally, the more we talk, the better I feel. But for the first time in my life, I didn't want discuss anything to do with fertility. Something inside me wanted to stay silent and shut.

Somehow, I know that if I let the words start pouring out, they are not going to be positive, productive words. They are going to be words of fear, of a foreboding that perhaps I am really not going to have another baby.

If I let the feelings that live inside my body form themselves into words, they are going to turn into words that drag my body down even further, maybe even permanently.

This time, I don't want to talk. I just want to win. I don't want to be comforted, soothed, or given advice.

I just want to win.

If I started in on a long discussion with Leah about having another baby, I would have to reveal how I am living off the faith that lives in my head. I would have to let it be known that I am ignoring the statistics, ignoring the facts, and creating my own reality based entirely on faith.

I am doing the most that medical science offers, but the bottom line is that I could not do this without believing in an alternative reality based on miracles and faith.

I pray God helps me have another baby, and I believe He will help me. I believe He wants my daughter to have a sibling to love.

I could tell Leah was hurt when I said that I did not want to talk about getting pregnant, but I just couldn't put into words the reality I am living right now.

Getting Ready for the Next IVF

I have my whole IVF planned. I am going to Dr. Deutsch three times next week. Once, the day before my eggs are retrieved. A second time the day before they are implanted, and then the day after they are implanted. Once I get pregnant (no ifs here) I am going to see him once a week to keep my body on track.

My husband hates the idea of traveling so far every week, but he hated the idea last time and look what happened.

Preparing to Conceive

Dr. Deutsch says I'm ready. He says my body is ready to conceive.

Eileen and I continue working on removing difficult memories from my body.

I have been getting my shots every night. When my husband gives me the shot, it is an oddly tender and tense time between us.

Sometimes, I adore him for his skill and experience in administering the shots. I love him for his ability to give the shots so quickly.

But if he pricks me or hits a wrong spot, I get super annoyed at him--like I think I would punch him if I could.

I am not making any plans because I expect to be pregnant soon all I want to do is incubate myself to help my baby survive.

Sunday Retrieval

Today was the egg retrieval.

We got to the hospital about 6 a.m. A kindly nurse at the desk welcomes us. For a moment, the whole place feels different—a fantasy island of fertility where surgical procedures are pink and beautiful. For a few minutes, I am lulled into actually believing this might turn out to be fun.

We were the ones on the floor that morning and we are put in a room at the end of the hallway. It is so quiet. I am not deceived by the wallpaper anymore. Now, it all feels very serious and very real, just like it did the other two times. I pray and pray. I always feel a measure of fear when I'm going under anesthesia. And heaviness. I feel a heaviness when it comes time to do an IVF, as if the weight of the world is on me.

Finally a young man comes to wheel me down to the OR. I have seen him before. He has wheeled me to several operations and procedures. He doesn't remember me, but I remember him. He must see a thousand like me each month.

In the waiting area, I am put me in front of station 3. Three? Could it mean..a sign that I am going to have triplets!!!!!

I let myself get a bit giddy imaging that this IVF will result in triplets. Triplets....Imagine! The instant large family of my dreams! My little girl suddenly blessed with three siblings! Three sisters? Oh my God, four girls!!!! Or maybe two girls and a boy? Oh my God, a family of three girls and one boy! Two boys and a girl? Then I would have two girls and two boys! Four children would be a lot of work at first, but my kids would never be lonely. I am imagining our family photo twenty years from now. All four kids and then someday all their kids will have babies and their kids will have lots and lots of cousins. In my old age, I'll always have a child to be with. I'll be busy with kids until I'm 58 years old!

I let this fantasy play out in my head and I am feeling happier and happier.

Triplets!

A few minutes later, I am wheeled into the operating room. The anesthesioligist is kind, and very quickly, I am asleep.

I wake up, I don't know how much later, in that horribly awlful waiting recovery area. But good news—I am told retrieved ten eggs! Ten! Oh my God! Ten!

All my hard work trying to get healthy paid off. I can't believe this. I probably will end up with six good eggs, and then there is a good chance that three of those six will take, and I will have triplets!

Can you imagine? My daughter will never be lonely. She will always have at least one sibling in the house to play with.

In three days, my eggs will be implanted back in me. Ten! I'm betting triplets are on the way!

Day of Transfer

Today was the transfer of the embryos, where they implant the eggs mixed with my husband's sperm back into me. I ended up with three eggs, not ten, but three.

Dr. M, the one who so devastated me a few months ago by saying my eggs were bottom of the barrel, was ironically, the doctor on hand for the procedure. As always during procedures, she was kind, generous and nurturing. I've figured out that she is good at handling tests, but not to have as the primary doctor on your case. Maybe she likes the non-pressure of just stepping in for a procedure, without the pressure of having to follow-up and figure out what is going on. Dr. M. said it was wonderful that I did everything the clinic asked of me, submitted to all the tests they recommended, including a balloon test known as a hysterosalpingogram that was not too pleasant. I just smiled, pretending to be laid back about the whole thing.

She never could have guessed how much she devastated me a few months ago. She seemed to have no anger or resentment over the fact that I dumped her and switched to another doctor. Maybe she is so busy, she didn't even notice that I had switched doctors at all. Or she was just relieved to be rid of a patient who was creating too much work for her.

Anyways, as she was just about to do the transfer, she said it was bad luck to have the same doctor do a transfer twice, especially since the last transfer she did didn't work out. So she went to get another doctor to insert my eggs. I was grateful for her sensitivity, especially since she was the one whose words made me feel so hopeless.

Before she went to get the other doctor, she took an ultrasound picture of my eggs and said, "Let's hope this is a first baby picture." Hopeful and kind words, and made me feel good. Imagine if this was my baby's first picture. She smiled kindly at me, and for a minute, I think I can forgive her for the pain she caused me.

The other doctor came in, did the transfer, and now I must wait and hope my baby comes soon.

Worn Out and Tired

It has been two days since the embryos were put into my body.

Most of the time, I am on my knees in prayer, asking God to send an angel to guide my embryos to life, to give this baby the breath of God. If He wants to empower my tired old eggs to turn into a baby, He can and will.

And I'm tired. So very tired.

Praying and Waiting

It is 5 o'clock in the morning. A light snow decorates the earth outside my window, and there are three embryos inside me fighting to live.

After changing doctors, eating according to blood type, taking two shots a day of some pretty powerful infertility drugs, going to acupuncture once a week, a myofascial release expert and a kinesiologist twice a month, I ended up with three fair-to-poor quality embryos.

If I have one baby, I will be glad. No, ecstatic. Overjoyed. Full of bliss and gratitude. Yet, there is a part of me who wants three babies, an instantly large family by today's standards.

I am trying not to be stressed. I am trying not to think negatively. I am trying not to hate myself, but right now, self-hate is roaring through my body. It seems no one in my life realizes how absolutely helpless you can feel when you've done everything medically possible both in conventional medicine and in alternative medicine and still end up with only three embryos.

Earlier this week, I made a collage representing pregnancy.

I got a giant poster-size paper and cut and glued pictures of babies and mothers and words like 'revel in your ripeness' 'miracle' 'prayers' and 'mom knows cool.' My collage is beautiful and I hung it in my office.

I love this collage. I look at it and think: 'it is possible. I could make a baby.'

For now, however, I'm going to cheer my little embryos on.

"Dear Embryos,

I don't know you yet. One of you, or all of you, may end up being one of the most important persons in my life. You may end up being the answer to my prayers. I may someday get to hold you and love you.

You may grow and become more than I ever imagined.
Right now, know I love you. I love you if you make it and I love you if you don't make it. I am cheering for you. I am trying to give you the best parts of me. I am your mother and you are my children, and I'm hoping we can take that connection into the physical realm. Take what you need to take from my body. Feed off me. Ignore my tired, cranky spirit. Ignore the self-hatred looming inside of me. Ignore all the mixed emotions that are stirring around in my head. Just hear this: you are loved. You are wanted. You will be given as much as I can give. Your sister Amber needs you. Your Daddy Chris is praying for your continued growth. I, your mother, sit nervously and tenuously, hoping Dec. 20 comes quickly and the answer is yes. Please, please, please, let the answer be yes."

I Am Pregnant

Today, I got the call: I am pregnant.

I was happy for a moment. Then I ran into the bathroom to check for blood.

The phone call came at 10 o'clock. When I got the news, I thought: "If I can make it to 5 o'clock with no blood, then I'll feel good."

Pregnant. For now. I keep going to the bathroom and checking

Tonight, I thought: one day down, nine months to go.

One Month Pregnant

It is January and I have been pregnant for a month.

I am happier than I would have been if I was not pregnant, but being just one month into my pregnancy, I live each day with fear and a bucket of sadness I can't shake.

Since the day I learned I was pregnant, I have not once gone to the bathroom without immediately checking for blood, holding my breath every time I wipe myself, and feeling waves of relief each time I see no blood.

I am ever vigilant about everything, from where I go, to what I eat, to how long I sit or stand. There are moments I feel relief, like Mondays when we go to the library storytime and visit my mother, or when I'm reading to my daughter and I sink into the in-love feeling I have for her, but other than that, my life feels very hard right now. I have a lot of faith, and a strong part of me feels that God would not have taken me this far to let me fall. If I did miscarry, I would never blame Him, nor would I give up.

I told Leah the other day that I feel weary in a way I never felt before.

When I visualize what is happening within me, I see a girl wearing an ugly brown vest over a once white and beautiful dress. She is laying on the floor and can't walk--she has no legs. She crawls instead and her hair is messy. This girl's inability to walk, in many ways, reflects how tired I feel, how completely worn down I am by the last few months events. This is in no way a relaxed, comfortable pregnancy. It is a pregnancy where I am crawling all the way to the finish line.

But there is another part of me. A woman who stalks the forest deliberately and carries my daughter on her back. She swings through trees, swims through rivers, and seems to be the one capable of doing the hard stuff now. She loves my little girl more than anything, and she keeps her on her back no matter what. She carries a knife, and will fight off bears, lions, anything that tries to get near her baby. It is a good feeling to visualize her now.

She doesn't seem as forlorn and scared as she once was.

Every week, we drive the hour and a half to Portland, Maine to see Dr. Deutsch. One week, he looked down at me with a very concerned expression and said, "it is good you came this week." He didn't say anymore and I thought: I wonder if he knows that if I didn't come, my body would have miscarried." Dr. Deutsch doesn't always say a lot, but I could sense by his tone that something serious was going on. As usual, he did his thing to strengthen my adrenals, thyroid, and whatever else was off whack, weak, or out of alignment. I thank God for this man's ability to help me.

He has become a key part of my journey this pregnancy.

April and Still Pregnant

It is April 6 and I am still pregnant. After almost two straight years of infertility hell for the second time around, I am now entering my fifth month of pregnancy.

I had mistakenly thought infertility hell would end the moment the nurse announced over the telephone that yes, I am pregnant.

But after so many disappointments, the hell only intensified: now I really had something I had to fight and pray to hold on to. Now I had something I could lose.

For a long time, it was a hell to hear that no, I was not pregnant, but a different type of hell ensued once the answer was yes. Now, a dream coming true is within my shaky reach, but could be yanked away by something crazy like poor egg quality or hormone imbalance.

So the hell has continued these five months...so much so, that I could barely write this journal. The first day I found out I was pregnant went by oh-so-slowly. I looked at the clock a million times. Was my baby still growing? Could I carry to term? Would I miscarry and start bleeding any minute? I remember looking at the clock that day at exactly 5 o'clock thinking: one day down, nine months to go.

I have not gone to the bathroom once during these past five months where I didn't hold my breath, look at the toilet paper for signs of blood, and at the blessed sign of no blood, say a quick prayer of thanks to God for helping my baby to survive.

The first month of pregnancy, intensified by high doses of progesterone shots adminstered every night, was an exercise in mental torment and hellish frustration. I woke up every night about midnight, and would stay wide awake until 4 or 5 o'clock.

I pray a lot. I pray very specifically: asking God to please, don't let me eat anything that could hurt my baby. Please, don't let me contract anything that could hurt my baby, like fifth disease. Please, please, please. Prayer is always at the tip of my lips.

It has been an odd pregnancy, not blissful like my daughter's, but fraught with the potential for great hurt. I feel like a young girl who has finally won the boyfriend of her dreams, only to know that the head cheerleader is after your guy, and no matter how hard you try, she is always right there smiling and tossing her wavy blonde pony tail.

In my third month of pregnancy, my wisdom tooth got infected, and I spent a few hysterical days imagining that the infection would kill my blossoming fetus. I tentatively went to the oral surgeon to have the tooth removed. Only, right before he was about to start, something inside me knew I shouldn't have this procedure. After much questioning, the oral surgeon finally admitted there were no guarantees that the novacaine would not hurt my baby.

I walked out. Pennicilon got rid of the infection and Dr. Deutsch agrees that I probably did the right thing in not having the tooth removed.

I found out last week I was having a boy, which brought with it a host of joyful feelings. I was ecstatic: me, having a boy, my old and tired body actually producing a boy.

Relief...Thanks...Amazement.....

My daughter speaks fondly of her brother, and often asks me why he can't come out now. "YES I WANT TO TAKE HIM OUT TOO" I want to tell her. I want to feel his beautiful cheeks against my cheeks and I want to kiss him and say thank you God, thank you baby, for finally arriving!!!"

I am on a medical leave from work, and it is tough not having this emotional outlet. I miss chocolate so much I dream about it. I have informed my husband that the moment Dr. Lirrette removes the baby from my body, that he is to present me with a box of Godiva chocolates, Mrs. Field's chocolate chip cookes and Chinese food (which I also can't have.)

I am also not allowed to eat a lot of fish, and I miss tuna fish. I often think longingly about a D'Angelo's tuna fish sandwich.

Yet, the other day at the ultrasound, I got a reward for all my discomfort: a large, beautiful, glossy ultrasound picture of my son.

My son...what marvelous words I thought I would never speak. He looked so cute! Adorable! Incredibly handsome like some Greek Adonis or something. The ultrasound technician, who was very kind, zoomed in to show me a close up of my son drinking my amniotic fluid.

When I saw his mouth moving, gulping in the fluid that Only my body is able to give him, my heart turned upside down and I fell crazy in love.

The day I found out I was having a boy, I looked in the mirror and for the first time in months, I felt pretty.

Don't ask me why, but I suddenly saw something different in myself that I hadn't seen for awhile.I don't know why finding out I was having a boy made me feel pretty, but I did.

Now I wait. Four and a half, perhaps five, months to go. I start the emotional training it will take to turn myself over to this little human who will need the best, kindest and most significant parts of me.

A journey has begun that I have needed for a very, very long time.

Today's Main Theme: Fear

Today is one of those days when fear seems to be the main theme running through my day.

Actually, I shouldn't say today is one of those days, when the reality is, during this pregnancy, every day is a day full of fear.

This morning, we went to the library with my mother for a story time and puppet show. Usually, this is one of my favorite times during the week. Yet today storytime wasn't so fun, because moments after we got to the library, I started to feel pain in my buttocks and with the pain came fear.

Lately any type of mild pain elicits fear in me. Pain: is something is wrong with my baby? Pain: (hell even mild discomfort)—am I about to lose my baby? Pain: Did I do something to hurt my baby?

So the rest of the time at the library, I asked my mother to watch my daughter. I sat down and didn't move, because I was afraid that too much movement would hurt my baby.

Tonight, I am left thinking: Was there ever a time in my life when my body was free to do what it wanted without fear? Was there really a time when I could move any way I wanted without worrying that I was moving too fast or too something?

After the library, we went to Friendly's, a favorite of my daughter. I desperately wanted the cheese quesadillas, but I read that soft cheese isn't safe during pregnancy, and although quesadillas are made with hard cheese, that information on soft cheese has made me very weary of cheese in general, and throughout this pregnancy, cheese has been something I eat with suspicion.

Another blow to freedom. I ate onion rings instead, as I am afraid to eat chicken, hamburger, or any type of meat at restaurants (what if they undercook the meat and that hurts my unborn child?)

I admit: I am paranoid. Had I had my babies in my 20s and never gone through infertility, I'm sure I would have heartily enjoyed cheese quesadillas and a hot fudge sundae today.

I am antsy. I am bored out of my mind. I want to stay up all night and drink wine with friends. I want to eat mounds of chocolate, piles of cheese quesadillas, and loads of hamburgers. I want to be able to go to the library on Monday, and run as wild and free as my daughter, and not for a minute worry about pulling a muscle or doing something to hurt my unborn baby.

Instead, it is 7:26 p.m. and I will probably be asleep in half an hour. I cherish this little boy inside me. So much so, I am a walking advertisement for what happens after lots of reproductive trauma, and so I forgive myself kindly and when this little boy arrives, I am going to smother him in an absurd number of kisses.

Then I am going to ask my husband to please pass the cheese quesadillas.

Wishing For Popcorn and Molasses

Right now, I want to the calendar to say 1982 again, and I'm back at my parents' house doing my homework on the couch as my mother surprises me with a big white plastic bowl of popcorn smothered in butter and molasses that she popped on our brown stove in a regular frying pan.

Last night, a horrible thunder and lightning storm ruined my evening.

Then today I had severe stomach pains and I thought something was wrong with my baby. I ended up going to see my ob/gyn for an ultrasound.

The baby was fine, thanks to God. Now I'm just tired, and craving the safety that once existed when I was young and able to eat my Mom's molasses and butter popcorn. Why does life have to turn out so hard sometimes?

June: Feeling Overwhelmed

It arrived in the mail the other day. The date for my caesarean has been scheduled. I'm not crazy about the date, and so when I go to my doctor this week, I might ask for another date. But seeing a definite date written on paper, scheduled in somebody's appointment book, makes me happier than one can imagine.

We have lots of ideas on how to help my daughter adjust to her new brother. We are going to buy her a beautiful, beautiful, beautiful (did I say beautiful?) dress and give it to her the morning of my caesarean so she can wear it to the hospital for her first official meeting with her brother.

We are also going to give her a gift a day for the first two weeks after the baby is born...wrapped with pretty paper and lots of bows.

Nothing too expensive mind you, but small things, like a book, a Barbie, maybe a game or two, a t-shirt that says, "I'm A Big Sister Now", a cake with a picture of her and her new little brother on it.

I want the day of his birth to arrive now.

Countdown to August. Here it comes...

Last Day of June

Today is the last day of June. In 52 days, my son will be born. I am moving closer and closer to that long awaited day of his birth, but I still feel like I am a 100 miles away from a much needed glass of water on a scorching July day.

I can't let myself relax into this pregnancy, can't let down my guard for a moment, because if I do, there is always the fear that something could go very wrong.

My life has gotten very small this pregnancy.

I don't go many places.

Sometimes, when I hear a song from my past, I start to cry: was there ever really a time in life when I was so free and without fear constantly accompanying me? It seems impossible.

These nine months have seemed like 20 years, slow, terrible, every step a warning. I don't feel normal very often anymore.

There have been joyous moments too. Each week, when I get my ultrasound, and see my son growing, surrounded by plenty of healthy placenta and fluid to keep him well-fed, I feel a slight relief.

Each time I leave Dr. Lirrette's office, I marvel that I was able to find such an outstanding doctor.

18 Days To Go

I am 18 days away from giving birth. It still feels like a million years from now, 20 years at least. A year when I'm feeling good.

I am still nervous. Still paranoid. Not as fearful as I was, say, six months ago, but still not as relaxed as I should be. I know the odds are in my favor, but still, I've never been one to find comfort in the odds.

I pray a lot. I pray that God protects me and my baby from fifth disease, bacterial poisoning, car accidents, listeria, anything and everything that could hurt my baby.

I am excited about my son's birth, but not fully comfortable allowing myself to feel happy just yet.

Countdown To My Son

I am in countdown mode. Two weeks until my scheduled c-section. It still feels like a million light years away.

This journey has been long, grueling, sometimes unbearable. It has included six IUIs, three IVFs, and 9/11 occuring the day before my second IVF.

Getting pregnant also included a weekly hour and a half drive to a chiropractor/kinesiologist, a weekly visit to an acupuncturist, several hundreds of dollars spent on homeopathy, visits to an herbal expert where I bought bags of herbs each week that had to be boiled into tea and hours and hours spent at the bookstore researching the topic of infertility.

Achieving this pregnancy also included having two shots a day in my thigh, stomach or butt for three weeks in preparation of my IVF cycle and progesterone shots that made me slightly crazy every day for six weeks once I became pregnant.

Could this hell really be almost over?

Even though I'm nearing the finish line, I feel safer keeping up my guard.

The other day, we went shopping at a big baby store and there was this little blue outfit that said, "Thank heaven for little boys." Just seeing those words made me start to cry.

When I got home, I started eating watermelon. Wham--without ten minutes, I was vomiting profusely, wondering where this vomit was coming from, since I felt no pain or nausea.

Of course, since this never happened to me before, I was scared and phoned Dr. Lirrette. The poor man must have cringed when he saw my name on the beeper, since at least once every two weeks I have gone in for an emergency appointment or called in because of this pain or that pain.

But being the great doctor he is, Dr. Lirrette called back within 10 minutes. All I can say is, thank God he is my doctor. Most doctors would have kicked me to the curb by now.

The rest of the night, I became whiny, asking my husband to please, go buy me an almond slush, please, please massage my back and legs, please, could he juice me some garlic and lemon (in case I had a stomach bug).

My daughter kept asking, "Mom, why do you like garlic lemonade so much?"

Two Hours To Take-Off

In two hours, I will be going to the hospital to have my c-section.

Two hours..have I really made it this far? I am still praying to God that nothing happen to my baby...can you imagine...even at this point, fear still looms. I feel undeserving of this miracle.

One would think by now I would feel at ease, full of hope that everything was going to be all right, and yet I am afraid to let myself be happy.

I am more than thankful that this nine months of hell is almost over.

Two hours. Did I really make it this far? Me? Me who usually messes up and fails?

Right now, so many emotions are churning inside me, from fear to worthlessness to awe.

I am waiting.

The Birth Of My Son

A month and three days ago, my son was born. It seems like forever and a day ago that I was wide awake at 2 a.m., waiting anxiously for morning so the birth of my son could begin...my darling prince could finally arrive.

Where do I start in flashing back to one of the most momentous and long-anticipated moments in my life.

To start, I am not the same person I was a month and three days ago.

Back then, I still boiled constantly with fear that something would go wrong and my son would not come to me.

August 22 began early for me. I was scheduled for my c-section at 7:30--ironically the same time as my daughter's c-section, and I could hardly wait for this day to get started.

Instead of being relaxed, I was still worried that something terrible would go wrong and take my baby away from me.

I was up the whole night before my son's birth, too excited to sleep, so excited for it all to begin, I did not want to miss a moment. I felt like I was waiting for this moment all of my life. A son! A son coming to me! Me! Actually me! I refused to sleep all night.

I would not be absent for a moment of this moment.

Finally, finally, 5 a.m. arrived and I could begin the day."Can you believe the day is here?" I whispered to my husband, who was still half asleep.

"You made it," my husband said.

"Don't say that," I cringed, still in fear that something might go wrong at the last minute. I loved him for trying to boost me up, but I didn't feel safe letting myself completely relax yet.

It was damp that morning, a slight chill in the air, surprising
after the long hot summer. I wanted to look beautiful to meet my son,
but I had avoided salons for nine months, because of fear of chemicals,
so my hair was long, unruly, a big knot in the back. I had tried to cut my
own hair about five months before, which resulted in an even bigger
mess. Still, I applied my make-up carefully, and put my hair up to hide
the mess it had become.

Now I was done showering, doing my make-up and hair. I put on the
purple top and shorts that was one of only three pregnancy outfits I
wore these past months.

The first day I learned I was pregnant, I spent the day checking myself in
the bathroom every hour to make sure I was not bleeding. To be in my
bedroom that morning, dressing to go the hospital with a
full living baby thriving inside me seemed almost too much, too good,
too impossible, to be true.

Then it was time to wake our daughter. We spent a lot of time thinking
about how we could make this transition easy on her. We bought her a
beautiful flowered white satin dress to wear to the hospital and several
new toys to be given to her over the next few weeks. "Honey, today is
the day your baby swims out," I said.

She smiled sleepily. We couldn't wait any longer, and we gave her the
first of her presents: an Enchanted Forest Barbie with storybook.

Now we were all dressed, and headed downstairs to be with my parents,
who had stayed over the night before. I took out my camera and was
snapping pictures of this and that, trying oh so hard to capture the
moments before my son arrived.

Like many mothers before me preparing for the moment of their baby's
birth, I knew I was stepping into one of life's timeless moments and I
wanted it all on film.

Then we drove to the hospital. Once inside, I went up to the third floor
maternity ward, the same one where my daughter was born.

I took a picture of my husband holding my daughter, standing next to my parents, going up in that elevator. Everyone looks serious, tired, happy. I love that picture.

At the hospital, I was escorted into a room to be prepped. The two nurses assigned to me were kind, funny, and nice. They had a hard time getting my IV in, but looking back, even the discomfort of the IV wasn't bad. I was lucky that my doctor, Dr. Lirrette, inserted the catheter that I was so dreading. He is a gentle and kind man, who I feel amazingly safe and comfortable with.

He was one of the few aspects of my pregnancy where I did feel completely safe. Every woman on earth preparing to give birth should be so fortunate as to have a doctor like Dr. Lirrette.

Then it was on to the operating room for the C-section. Dr. Lirrette walked me and my husband down to the room.

My husband had to leave for the epidural. During the epidural, Dr. Lirrette held my hand to get me through it and kept saying things like, "You can do it" and "You're the best" and "think of your beautiful baby" in such a confident and gentle way that the epidural barely hurt. In fact, I can't even remember it because Dr. Lirrette's reassuring voice overshadowed any fear or pain in that moment.

But once the epidural was done, another drama had begun. I was numb--even my mouth was numb. People were running in and out of the OR. Time seemed to drag on. I was so nervous.

"Why do you like playing cards?" I asked my husband, because I wanted to distract myself, as my stomach was being cut open. I waited for what seemed like a long, long time.

"Paula, look, the baby is here," Dr. Lirrette called out.

"I can't look," I said, in fear that if I looked, I would see my cut-open stomach.

'Look!" and the sheet came down and I could see the very long umbilical cord attached to this golden beautiful boy. My boy...my boy....here.

It was all so surreal, that even now I can't totally focus on that moment without a fuzzy blur of heaven opening up and my son coming to me surrounded by clouds of white. It was almost like a light surrounded my son, a culmination of a dream that I didn't feel totally deserving of and still doubted even when the reality hit.

I looked at him, and thought, "He looks like an angel...he looks just like an angel." He was golden, completely golden, and perfect.

Then he was ushered away for shots and a clean-up, and I was on my way to recovery.

A few minutes later, in the recovery room my parents came in with my daughter.

"He looks strong honey," my father said.

Then I went to my room, and waited for what seemed like hours for the nurse to bring my son.

During those first moments together with my son I remember only two things: he was beautiful and I immediately liked his personality. I sensed a goodness and kindness about him. I remember him rooting immediately, and staring at me, as if playing that tape to him each night with my voice paid off, because he seemed to recognize my voice. I was surprised that he wanted to breast feed so easily and so soon.

So much happened during those five days in the hospital...there are flashes of memories that come and go..me ordering chocolate cake from the cafeteria, delighted that finally I could eat chocolate again...my daughter crying hysterically on the last night of my stay at the hospital that she missed me...me breast feeding in front of visitors and not at all caring who saw my breasts and me feeling incredibly proud that my son wanted so desperately to drink milk from my tired and sagging old breasts.

There is one particular incident, however, that best summed up my son's birth.

Two days after my son was born, a cafeteria worker found my son's alarm on the floor. The alarm on my son's leg that was suppose to protect him from being abducted had fallen off. To say I was upset was an understatement, and the more I tried to get an explanation, the more the nurses, aides and everybody else went into defensive mode. They insisted security was not violated, and I insisted that it was.

"Could someone have walked off this floor with my baby?" I wanted to know.

"No," they insisted. I didn't buy their explanation.

Night came, and I was still feeling scared, restless, full of trepidation that I had come so far, delivered a healthy baby, only to lose him somehow at the hospital because of a security glitch. I almost checked out of the hospital early because of fear that security at the hospital was poor. All kinds of scary scenarios played out in my head. My husband insisted we stay, which probably was for the best, but I still felt uneasy.

Around 8 o'clock, I started missing my son terribly. The nursery was a long walk down the hallway, but I decided I was going to see him regardless. Walking was still hard for me. Any movement at all was hard and I was in great pain, but I kept walking. I'd inch a few feet, stop, inch a few more.

I finally got to the nursery, wearing a blood-stained nightgown, but not really caring that I was a mess.

I walked in the nursery, took one look at my son in his incubator, and burst out crying. I hated him being away from me. I hated that I was too weak to care for him at night.

"I just miss him so much," I said. "I am so worried that he's not safe."

The nurses were cold to me, one even saying I must be hormonal because it was my third day after birth.

My guess is that they feared getting in trouble over the missing alarm. I hobbled back to my room, sad, but proud that I had forced myself down that long hallway to see my son. He was here, a part of who I was, and there was no turning back.

That image of myself; a ragged, disheveled woman, wearing a blood-stained night gown, and who looked like a neurotic mess and probably was a bit over the top, is who I am most proud of. She was the mother warrior who walked me through the years of infertility treatments, who dared to defy the doctor who said the game was over and no more children would be coming to me because of my old and dwindling number of eggs.

It was that crazy lady who dragged herself to appointment after appointment, test after test, and who tried everything from homeopathy to acupuncture, to get this much desired baby. And in that craziness, in that mother lion, was a strength, a love, and a complete willingness to look like a fool if it would someday bring my beloved child to life.

Only a nut keeps trying when it looks hopeless...only a nut..and so if the nurses thought me a bit quirky and weird, so be it. If the only way I could arrive at the nursery to see my son was to hobble down the hallway wearing a very icky blood-stained night gown because I was too tired to change, so be it.

Today I hold my son and he is here. Crazy nuts who do not give up are sometimes not so crazy. Prayers are indeed answered. Thank you Father in heaven. Amen.

The Beginning: A New Journey Has Begun

I am now a mother of two children. I say these words with pride, trepidation, and a feeling that unless you've gone through infertility, it is a statement that could sound deceptively ordinary and mundane.

Two children, 'that's nice, so what', could be the reaction of someone whose children arrived unexpectedly, without much effort or planning, after a wonderful night or two of love making.

But for a woman who has endured four years of infertility treatments, 16 IUIs, four IVFs, two shots a day month after month, and who once put two chocolate donuts on her stomach as an incentive to get her through a painful test, being able to say she has two children is perhaps the most amazing, the most momentous achievement one can imagine.

I might have well been elected the first female president, or climbed Mount Everest, or written 'Gone with the Wind'.

For someone like me, being able to say I have two children is like being able to say that your craziest, wildest, most important dream actually came true.

I might have well won ten million dollars, or flown to the moon alone, or found the cure that would have allowed Christopher Reeve to walk.

Something that seems so regular and so ordinary is anything but ordinary to me, and that is both the beauty of suffering with infertility and the curse of suffering with it.

I cherish my children in a way that is slightly different, because I know from bitter experience how tough it can sometimes be for a sperm and egg to successfully join together and make it through the nine months to transform into a healthy baby.

I've seen science up close, in a way I sometimes wish I never saw it, but in a way that makes every new baby I see seem like the greatest invention ever.

I sometimes look at my children, during the most ordinary of moments, and I think, "Good God, it all worked out. Somehow, it all worked out."

And often, in those moments, I feel a sort of survivors' guilt, because I know for many women, it doesn't work out, and I get angry and sad all at once. I want to tell them 'don't give up! never give up hope!

Don't listen to the doctors who tell you your eggs are too old' don't listen to well-meaning friends and relatives who say crazy, stupid things like, "maybe God doesn't want you to have a child." I want them to know that infertility is not a result of being flawed in some way, or cursed in some way, but it is a sickness, a disease, just like breast cancer, heart disease or the common cold.

It is a physical problem, and sometimes all the relaxing in the world won't make a baby.

When I look back, over the past five years, and I analyze closely the step-by-step process of getting pregnant, staying pregnant, and giving birth, I get depressed and then tired. It was too much. Too hard, too long, too painful--and thank God I didn't know that at the time and thank God I experienced all of it. Thankfully, as I walked that road, I never knew how long and how hard it would be. As a young teen, I learned the poem, "inch by inch, life's a cinch. Yard by yard, it is hard. Mile by mile, it is a trial" and sometimes when everything got too hard I'd say to myself, 'inch by inch' and I kept slowly inching forward towards my goal.

At one point, when I so desired my second baby, I would wake up each day, open my appointment book, and write a list of what I could do that day to move me closer to my goal. Sometimes it was doing things like eating lots of salad, avoiding coffee, or making an appointment with my acupuncturist.

Sometimes it meant going to swimming, listening to my relaxation tapes, and of course praying. Always praying. I was a woman at war, and every day I had to pull together my strategy.

Now I am a mother. A new journey has started for me.

I have the little girl I yearned for, and the son that I so wanted to complete my family.

My daughter is not an only child, and in seeing her with a brother, I see all the advantages I had being the only one, and all the disadvantages I had.

It has made me cherish my childhood even more, and at the same time, I am profoundly thankful that their lessons will be different than mine. What has the experience with infertility taught me? First, on a practical level, I firmly believe that infertility clinics should be taking advantage of all that is offered by holistic and alternative practitioners. Sadly, eastern and western medicine refuse to come together. Holistic practitioners often discount the power and effectiveness of conventional medicine.

Some of the holistic and alternative practitioners I worked with recommended that I stop using the medicines and techniques available at the infertility clinic. Had I listened to them, I doubt my two children would be here today. Conventional medicine has made great and daunting strides in helping women have children, and to not take advantage of all the science available would be foolish. I know that without the IUIs and the IVFs and all the medication I took, my children would not be here. To not tap into these powerful medications and procedures would have probably meant not meeting the two most awesome people I ever imagined.

At the same time, there no denying that there is a lot that alternative medicine has to offer, as it can sometimes uncover the subtle reasons, not so easily detected on standard tests, why a woman is having a problem getting pregnant, reasons that conventional doctors all too easily label and dismiss as 'unexplained infertility.' There are millions of women who can't get pregnant for specific reasons never uncovered by conventional medicine. There are also millions of women who miscarry again and again, and no explanation is offered.

Alternative medicine delves into these murky, difficult-to-understand areas.

It looks at things like the impact of emotions on a women's reproductive system, the condition of the adrenal glands, thyroid, kidney and liver that can impact conception and pregnancy, and the role nutrition may play in the body's readiness to conceive. My question is: why isn't acupuncture available at all the infertility clinics as part of the treatments, as a compliment to standard treatment?

Why aren't women undergoing infertility treatments told to stop the coffee, cut out the white flour and sugar, and get themselves on a healthy diet? Why do infertility clinics allow coffee to be served in their waiting rooms?

Why isn't there a massage therapist available to stressed out infertility patients--especially before procedures like IVF and IUI, as a means of helping patients relax?

Isn't it time that alternative medicine and conventional medicine come together to help struggling infertility patients. The two should not see each other as the enemy. I would be willing to say that many more women could successfully have babies if conventional infertility treatments and alternative medicine joined together.

 Isn't it time the battle over infertility be fought on all grounds--rather than two opposing teams who really need to be allies.

I know that this experience took away a feeling of carefreeness I once had. I'm more cautious, more serious, wounds leftover from a lady scarred in the battle, but somehow one who survived this fertility war.

I am stronger now, different, even thankful for this tumultuous and sometimes painful journey. It molded and sculpted me into a mother and was probably the best preparation for parenthood I could have asked for.

My journey now is using what I learned to help others, and somehow putting it all to good use as a mother. I'll remember the words of my dear friend Chelsea Lowe, who said, "For some women, this comes easily. For you, it is a long and difficult road.

It doesn't mean you can't eventually have what others have, but it does mean you have to travel down a different road."

So I walked that road, unfair as it was, and I came to the destination that many women ultimately come to: I am a mother.

Amazing.

The walk was hell, but oh, the destination sweet.

A Bonus Excerpt from Dancing Your Way to Fertility available on Amazon.com and at www.dancingyourwaytofertility.com.

Infertility: A Training Ground for Motherhood?

In times past, women have always endured sacrifice and trial as part of motherhood. Now, due to a host of factors such as age, health and environment, women are put through a severe test of their maternal stamina even before they conceive their child.

This road, this test, this initiation, will test all of you--and it will make you one of the strongest, most capable, confident, resourceful, perseverant mothers a child could ever have. Experiencing infertility gives you a lifetime pass to enjoy motherhood in a way few ever get to enjoy it, because with the difficulties of this disease come confidence and appreciation.

This journey will demand all the best parts of you. It will demand you persevere when you want to give up.

It will demand patience and persistence when frustration and helpless surrender might feel like a more natural path.
It will demand that every survival skill you possess be brought forth and utilized. It will demand sacrifice, self-preservation, and a willpower beyond what you knew you had, but what intrinsically you knew you were capable of.

If you are not fortunate, you may have your heart broken in 1000 pieces.

If you are fortunate, you could still have your heart broken in 1000 places.

When you give birth to your baby none of it will matter. Your heart will heal, the scars will seem insignificant, and all the tears, disappointments and devastations will seem like bunny rabbits and balloons on a summer's day.

No big deal.

If you do not give birth to a baby, but decide to adopt, become a foster parent, a teacher, coach, counselor or play a very active role in the life of a young niece, nephew, neighbor, or cousin, you will be ready and able to mother these children and impact a younger generation in a way more powerful than you ever imagined.

You have probably been through the best training course for motherhood possible: you understand pain, you understand the potential for joy, you are willing to do the work to get the child you want, and you've proven you can take the bad stuff that comes with going after the good stuff. In doing this, you will join a group of super cultivated mothers, women ready to nurture and love the next generation, and have more than proven their worth to do this.

Infertility hurts.

Winning over infertility can be a painful process that demands resolve and sacrifice.

It is an initiation rite, of sorts, an involuntary one, of course.

No one should have to go through this to have a baby and no one would voluntarily choose this road. Nonetheless, it is a reality for many of us, and it will prepare you for motherhood in a grand and inspiring way that someday you may even feel thankful to have experienced.

It is a long road and an unfair one, but at the end of the road, you could be holding the baby of your dreams, just as the same as someone who made love one night and woke up pregnant the next morning.

Then nothing at all will matter but your baby.

12 Cleanses To Help Restore Your Fertility

A Bonus Excerpt from Dancing Your Way to Fertility available on Amazon.com and at <u>www.dancingyourwaytofertility.com</u>.

The next step in changing the state, or condition, of your body is cleansing and detoxifying. The importance of detoxifying your body should never be underestimated. In this chapter, we'll look at 12 cleanses that can help restore and maximize your fertility potential.

Please note: cleanses should be done before you start infertility medications or treatments, because you do not want them to interfere with medications or a pregnancy, if there is even a slight chance you could be pregnant. Cleansing can be compared to overturning and fertilizing the soil before planting the seed.

If you are just starting infertility treatments, you may want to choose just one or two cleanses, so as not to delay treatment.

If you've been trying to get pregnant for a long time with no success, you might want to consider doing various cleanses to strengthen your body.
Here are some cleanses to consider:

• A Liver Cleanse

Never never NEVER underestimate the importance of having your liver cleaned and detoxified. The liver is a highly influential organ that plays a key role in fertility and is one of the most important organs in your body.

The liver governs approximately 500 metabolic processes and many studies have shown that the oestrogen receptors in the liver are critical for maintaining fertility.

I cannot say enough about the importance of having a clean, de-toxified liver in the quest to get pregnant.

An ineffective liver allows toxins to seep into the ovaries and endocrine system.

If your liver is congested, it cannot adequately remove toxins and fats from the body.

Instead, they will continue to recirculate through your system—causing hormonal disturbances and imbalances. It also means your ovaries will be flooded with toxic substances that your liver was suppose to clean—and your ovaries are the source of your eggs. These impurities will result in poor egg quality—all because your liver was too congested to do its job. So if you want to improve the quality of your eggs, make sure your liver is as clean and detoxified as possible.

Once the liver is cleansed, the entire endocrine and reproductive system becomes free of toxins and impurities, so they can begin functioning at a higher capacity.

What causes a sluggish, tired liver? Stress, poor diet, medication, toxins in the environment, low-quality food, coffee, sugar, white flour products and low quality drinking water, are among a few of the culprits. The older we get, the more our liver needs to be cleaned out because of the junk that we have taken into our body over the years.

A liver cleanse will help kick your body into high gear, increasing energy and vitality to all your organs.

Liver cleanses can be found online and at most health and natural food stores.

You may want to do a 30-day cleanse more than once. Please note: A liver cleanse should never be done while you are taking infertility medications, as it could interfere with the effectiveness of the medication. It is something to do BEFORE you begin any infertility treatments or medication, and is never to be done if you could be pregnant.

In addition to a liver cleanse, here are some other ways to detoxify, cleanse and strengthen your liver:

• Milk thistle is a wonderful herb for cleansing the liver. Read the directions on the bottle carefully as to amounts taken.

• Lemon is a great liver cleanser. About 20 minutes before breakfast in the morning, squeeze the juice from one or two fresh lemons into some warm water and drink.

• Beets are excellent liver cleansers. You can eat them cooked or juice them. To juice beets, peel and cut into small wedges that can easily fit in your juicer. Juice the beets with some apple, spinach or kale.

• Chlorophyll is a highly esteemed liver cleanser.

• Artichokes are powerful liver protectors because they contain a flavonoid called silymarin, which is an antioxidant that protects the liver from toxicity.

• Foods that are good for your liver include: spirulina, garlic, carrots, romaine lettuce, apples, grapefruit, chicory, mustard greens, dandelion greens, avocados, walnuts, turmeric and parsley.

• Cabbage can also be juiced and is effective in cleaning the liver.

• Amino acids, derived from healthy sources of protein, are key to the liver working at maximum capacity. Foods that contain these amino acids include: nuts, such as pumpkin seeds, squash seeds and almonds; lean meats, eggs, and beans, such as lentils and garbanzo.

• In Chinese medicine, infertility is often linked to Liver chi stagnation, a result of stress, overwork, and the effects of coffee and alcohol. Irritability, headaches and frustration are just some of the physical and emotional symptoms of liver chi stagnation. Acupuncturists and herbalists can work on unblocking energy stagnation in the liver.

• According to Chinese medicine, emotional and lifestyle cures for liver stagnation include being assertive, making clear decisions and enjoying lots of fun, laughter and relaxation. Holding on to anger, feeling stuck and depression impair the liver by stagnating the energy. Letting go, moving on, and exercising control over one's life, can help in healing the liver.

For more cleanses, visit DancingYourWayToFertility.com or Amazon.com.

How to Improve Your Egg Quality

A Bonus Excerpt from Dancing Your Way to Fertility available on Amazon.com and at <u>www.dancingyourwaytofertility.com</u>.

Good news—you can improve the health and quality of your eggs.

In the past, we were told we were all born with a certain number of egg cells that run out as we age. We were led to believe that egg cells were the only cells in the body that did not regenerate, but instead were a finite number. We are finding out THIS IS JUST NOT TRUE. Recent research has shown that women can produce new eggs throughout their reproductive years.

You may have been told that your eggs are not healthy or that your eggs are too old.

Here's the great news: there is much you can do to enhance the health of your eggs.

It was commonly believed that the only factor that determined egg health and quality was age. Several new studies have shown that stress, hormones and environmental toxins all impact our egg health.

Your egg's health is a key cornerstone of a healthy fertility, because the health of your eggs can affect whether or not fertilization, implantation and ultimately a healthy pregnancy and birth will occur.

Here are some things you can do to improve your egg health:

• Coenzyme Q10: Coenzyme Q10 is an excellent way to improve the quality and energy within your eggs.

In several studies, the supplement Coenzyme Q10 has been shown to improve egg quality.

It boosts energy production in the oocytes, which are cells in the ovary. Providing additional energy in the form of Coenzyme Q10 is needed when there is decreased energy production in the ovaries due to aging.

It is also a source of fuel for the mitochondria, which produces energy within the cells and with age, can begin to weaken. Along with taking a Coenzyme Q10 supplement, natural sources of CoQ10 include almonds, spinach, sardines, broccoli, strawberries, and walnuts.

For more on egg health, Dancing Your Way to Fertility is available on Amazon.com or visit www.dancingyourwaytofertility.com.

The People In Your Journey and Some of the Rude Comments You May Hear Along the Way

A Bonus Excerpt from Dancing Your Way to Fertility available on Amazon.com and at www.dancingyourwaytofertility.com.

This is not to be misinterpreted as an exercise in dumping family or friends, because people are not perfect and we should not expect them to be, and there are people in our lives, as unpleasant as they may be, that we simply need to forgive, stay connected to and be around.

Despite their flaws, we owe them something. That being said, as you walk this journey, you need to be ready for some of the stupid, rude and totally insensitive comments you are going to hear. Sometimes, people you love will say really dumb things.

Other times, it could be a stranger who zaps you with a statement that leaves you breathless and feeling punched in the gut.

Here are a few of the stupid, rude, thoughtless and COMPLETELY FALSE comments you may have to deal with, and how best to respond:

• **"Maybe you weren't meant to have a baby":** Yes, you were meant to have a baby. Yes, you were.

Millions of women have babies whether they want them or not, whether they will be good mothers or not, so why shouldn't you have a baby? In fact, there is NOT ONE REASON IN THIS UNIVERSE why you should not have a baby.

This person is either jealous of you or just likes to pop the balloon of hope. People who mouth off a comment like this mistakenly feel they have some sort of moral authority. Ignore them. They are wrong. Completely and utterly wrong.

• **"Aren't you a little too old to be trying for a baby?"**

Whoever got the idea that a young mother is better than an older mother has not seen the millions of mothers in their 40s and even 50s who mother with great patience, love, insight, wisdom and kindness.

This person obviously doesn't understand that with age comes maturity and wisdom.

Someone who makes a comment like this may be focusing on the energy level of children, forgetting that even most 25 year old mothers are not out playing baseball with their kids everyday.

Whoever throws out a comment about age is ignorant of the fact that a woman of any age who is ready and able to love a child, and who is brave and strong enough to endure infertility, is more prepared, capable and ready to mother than almost anyone. A good mother is a good mother, whether she is 21, 31, 41, 51 or beyond.

Letting Go Of the Secret Thoughts and Hidden Beliefs That Might be Holding You Back from Getting Pregnant

A Bonus Excerpt from Dancing Your Way to Fertility available on Amazon.com and at <u>www.dancingyourwaytofertility.com</u>.

You may find this hard to believe, but hidden within your subconscious could be some negative perceptions of pregnancy, childbirth and motherhood that are holding you back from having a baby, without you even knowing it.

You may have some hidden fears or beliefs about becoming a mother that conflict with your desire to have a baby.

Sometimes, the body can hold two very different desires at once. One part of us wants one thing, another part of us wants another.

Consciously, you may want to become a mother more than anything in the world. Subconsciously, you may have fears that are making it hard for your conscious wishes to come true. These two very different parts of you could be playing a tug of war: who will win? Who will get their way? Whose needs will be met? This conflict can make it hard for us to really commit and do the work needed to get what we want.

This tug of war steals energy away from what your body really needs to be doing—and that is healing and getting pregnant.

Ultimately, the goal should be that all the different parts of you are working harmoniously together and have the same goal: to conceive a baby.

Deep fears and childhood issues sometimes need to be acknowledged, listened to and healed so you can move forward in having a child.

It is important that you discover and acknowledge all your feelings and beliefs about becoming a mother—even the ones that are not all warm and fuzzy. Our conscious self might want something, but if our subconscious does not want it, it could be off doing a dance of its own.

If your subconscious doesn't want something, your body could follow suit.

Subconscious fears about pregnancy, child birth or raising a child could even at times influence your hormones and the physical processes required for conception.

Does having doubt, fear, or hesitance about having children mean you won't be a great mother? Not at all. Millions of great Moms once had doubts or fears about becoming a mother. Millions more worried about pregnancy, childbirth and how their life would change. Embarking on a new life path naturally brings up feelings of doubt and fear.

To find out what your subconscious really thinks about getting having a child, start by asking yourself what you think about becoming a mother, and then write down whatever response comes from you without editing yourself. Allow your subconscious to voice its feelings on the subject without judgment or criticism.

Negative feelings or beliefs left unexpressed or unresolved hold considerable energy which can block conception. If you ignore your subconscious, it might stage a rebellion within your body—not allowing you to get pregnant because it wasn't given the respect and attention it deserved.

Begin by writing: "I will become pregnant soon" or "My womb is ready to receive" and then after you write that, start writing whatever comes up from deep within.

Let whatever comes up from within you come up, come out and be heard. Write without editing or judging what you are writing.

Do not consciously think about what is coming up, or try to force something you don't really feel or think. Just write.

This exercise can help you uncover what you are feeling about your infertility on many levels. It can also reveal if there is a part of you that wants to sabotage your efforts to become pregnant, or feels that you are not worthy of a baby. By knowing your innermost feelings, you can then work on bringing together the different emotions within you, so that you can achieve your goal. Later on, reread what you wrote and thank your subconscious for opening up.

Try not to judge your subconscious, even if what comes up is not exactly what you want to hear.

You could also write down the words: 'I deserve to have a baby' and then type or handwrite whatever comes up. Remember: No judging. No editing. No thinking this out. Write without restraint and let your deep internal self say what it needs to say.

Other writing prompts include:

• My body is ready to conceive and give birth to a baby
• It is safe to have a baby
• I deserve to have a baby
• I am good enough to be a mother and give birth to a baby
• My body is capable of giving birth
• A woman like me deserves to be a mother
• I am ready to be a mother and have children
• It is safe for me to become a mother
• Being a mother is a good thing for me

Honestly listening to every part of yourself shows your courage, because you are not going into denial.

Every part of you needs deserves to be listened to so they can all work together. If you ignore the needs of your subconscious, it could sabotage all the hard work you are doing to get pregnant.

Here are some questions to ask yourself, write responses to, and spend some time thinking about.

• **Are you afraid of repeating the same mistakes your parents made?:** Do you fear repeating some of the negative and dysfunctional family patterns you grew up with? Do you sometimes find yourself thinking, 'when I become a parent, I never want to do to my child what my parents did to me' or 'I never want to put my kids through what my parents put me through.'

• **Are you scared of becoming a mother?:** Do you have fears about becoming a mother, such as or 'I'm afraid of who I will become when I have a child' or 'I'm afraid I don't have what it takes to be a good Mom' or 'I'm afraid I won't be able to care for my child properly.'

• **Are you worried about losing some of your me-time once you have a baby?:** Are there aspects of your life that you really like that you are worried you will lose once you have a baby?

• **Do you fear that once you become a mother, you will turn into your own mother?:** Did your Mom behave or act in a way that you don't want to repeat and hurt you a lot as a child? Or did your Mom do things that you promised yourself you would never do? Did you long ago make a silent pact with yourself that you would never become your mother?

• **Do you sometimes feel infertility is a deserved punishment, either from yourself or from God, for something you've done or didn't do, in the past?:** Could infertility be something you think you deserve to suffer? Did you do something, or not do something, you believe merits you being infertile?

• **Do you feel God is mad at you?:** Do you feel God is judging you harshly for something you did in your past that you still feel guilty about?

• **Were you a victim of physical, sexual abuse or emotional abuse? Did you have an abusive parent?:** Do you ever fear that you will become an abusive parent like they were? If so, you might fear repeating negative family patterns.

• **Did you ever experience a trauma that has left you feeling unsafe and weary of new experiences?:** Are you open to new experiences or does doing something for the first time unnerve you? Do you often feel scared and worried about your safety?

• **Are you a bit of a control freak?:** Do you need to control everything in your life? Or are you able to let life flow naturally towards you?

Does the idea of having a baby make you feel too out of control? letting life happen is not something you are comfortable with?

• **Do you feel you really deserve a baby?:** Or do you feel unworthy of this joy? Is there something about who you are, or what you have done or experienced in life, that makes you think someone like you doesn't deserve a baby? Do you feel worthy of getting what you want?

• **Does yearning for something feel more natural and comfortable than actually getting what you want?:** Have you spent a lot of your life yearning? Are you the type of person who feels more comfortable when you are yearning, wanting or suffering over something you can't have?

• **Are you more comfortable when you are the one giving, rather than the one receiving?:** Do things like getting a gift or a compliment make you feel uncomfortable? Are you in the habit of being able to be on the receiving end of things?

For more of this chapter, visit DancingYourWaytoFertility.com or Amazon.com to purchase this book.

50 Creative Projects To Help You Tap Into Your Fertility

A Bonus Excerpt from Dancing Your Way to Fertility available on Amazon.com and at <u>www.dancingyourwaytofertility.com</u>.

Creativity is a powerful anecdote to feelings of hopelessness and depression. Doing creative activities can help you unlock and release negative energy patterns and paths in the body. Tapping into your creativity can help you transcend emotional blockages that may exist within your body.

Exploring your creativity can relax you, de-stress you, and give your body a dose of happy, healthy chemicals that can assist in healing infertility. Here are some creative exercises and activities to try while undergoing infertility treatments:

1. Make a collage representing birth, babies, and the body's ability to conceive and have a baby.

You'll need a poster board, construction paper, or whatever kind of paper feels right to you. Cut out pictures from magazines, books, newspapers, or download and print pictures from the Internet of babies, pregnant women, along with images and words that represent what getting pregnant and having a baby means to you. Then, glue them in whatever pattern you choose on the paper or poster board of your choice.

When I was trying to get pregnant with my second child, I made a huge collage that affirmed my body's ability to get pregnant. I cut out pictures of babies and words like "the princess has arrived" and "mother love."

I used lots of positive words that meant a lot to me and I personally connected to having children.

My collage had pictures that represented new life emerging and the upcoming and most definite arrival of my child. I hung it in my office so I could look at it and feed off its positive energy every day.

Making this collage was a very joyful experience for me, because I had been trying for over a year to get pregnant and was not successful. I was extremely depressed, but while making the collage, I entered a very optimistic and hopeful state of mind. Every time I looked at my collage, I felt renewed hope and a surge of power—something that I needed desperately to gain back at that time. A few months later, I did become pregnant and gave birth to my beautiful son.

So, collage away. I used a huge poster board which I felt made my collage something powerful to look at. Make sure to use whatever images, pictures, words strike a personal note for you.

2. **Make a collage celebrating babies.** Cut out photos of babies from magazines and write something at the top like: Welcoming All Babies— Including Mine! Or: Welcome To All The Babies and My Baby Too! Put a picture of yourself in the middle of this collage along with something that represents your baby's arrival. In doing this, you'll be setting out the welcome mat for your baby's arrival and reminding yourself that babies are born everyday and soon yours will be too!

3. **Make a collage on the topic of fertility.** Use words and pictures that represent your body enjoying a healthy state of fertility. If you see pictures that symbolizes fertility to you, add it to your collage. Make sure to put a picture of yourself in the middle of the collage, with words like: "My Body is Fertile" or "The World Around Me Is Fertile and I Am Fertile Too" or "I Am Part of A Fertile World." Surround your picture with powerful and meaningful images of fertility that you can personally relate to.

4. **Create a scrapbook titled "My Successful Journey To Motherhood"** and include in it whatever pictures, quotes, experiences or items reflect your story of having children.

5. **Go to a crafts store and purchase pink and blue buckets and make flower arrangements that you will have in your hospital room when you have a baby.** Get flowers and decorations that you want in your room when you have a baby.

6. **Play inspiring music, like the theme to the movie 'Rocky', and march around your living room, picturing your ovaries turning out a healthy baby.** Play music that puts you in a state of positive expectation and joy. Allow the music to help you transcend all doubt, if even for just a few minutes. Let the music carry you into a state of being where you allow yourself to feel your dream of being a mother coming true. Play a song that represents triumph and victory as you see yourself giving birth and becoming a mother. Then, as you play this song, move, march, dance in a celebratory way that says: my baby is on the way to me soon.

7. **Make a collage of all the goals and dreams in your life that came true, as a hefty reminder that good things do happen to you and will happen to you again.**

By reminding yourself that you can get what you want, you'll be triggering the thought of 'it happened once, it can happen again.' Along with words and images of goals and dreams that came true, include a picture of yourself next to a baby and write on the collage, "my dream of having a baby is my next dream about to come true." Hang it in a place where you can see it often.

8. **Write a song about your victory over infertility.** Songwriting is a way to express your feelings about having a baby in a hopeful and positive way. Write and sing a song about the triumphant way your body was able to conceive and give birth to a baby, as if it already happened. Write a song inviting your baby to find a home in your womb. Write a song to your future child about all the wonderful things you will do together. You don't have to be musically inclined to pen a song that speaks of hope and the happiness that awaits you.

9. **Cut out words that describe the strength of your body and glue them onto a large piece of poster paper.** Put a picture of yourself in the center of these words, which can include words like: Fertile. Reproducing. Wise. Strong. Healthy. Ripe. Hang it somewhere where you can look at it often.

10. **Imagine you are a coach and let your inner fertility coach give you tips on how to get pregnant.** See getting pregnant as a game and listen to what your inner coach has to say about what you need to do to win this game. You can ask your inner coach to create a playbook, with what 'plays' or actions need to be taken for you to win at this fertility game. Draw a picture of your inner fertility coach and write down your inner coach's five best pieces of advice, and hang it somewhere you can see it often.

You know more than you think and this is one way to tap into that inner knowing.

All 50 creative exercises are available in Dancing Your Way to Fertility, available on Amazon.com.

Letters To Yourself

A Bonus Excerpt from Dancing Your Way to Fertility available on Amazon.com and at <u>www.dancingyourwaytofertility.com</u>.

During your fertility journey, there are times you will need to be your own best friend. Here are some letters that you can mail to yourself, or leave around the house when you need a lift or just a reminder of how strong you are. Be sure to begin each letter by filling in your name and then signing it at the end.

Dear_____

Congratulations! You are on your way to getting pregnant! Every day, you are one step closer to being pregnant! Every day, your body is getting stronger. I see you getting stronger! I can feel how ready your body is to conceive a baby. You are ready to have a baby! That's right-- your body can easily have a baby now! Congratulations!
Love,

Dear _____

I know with all my heart that you will give birth to a baby soon. Your dear sweet ovaries, dear healthy healthy ovaries, can produce ripe, rich healthy eggs. Actually, right now they are making healthy fertile eggs! Your ovaries know how to produce good eggs. They are right now producing eggs that will lovingly grow into your baby. Thank you ovaries! Thank you for giving me healthy eggs!

Love,

_____

Dear_____:

You are ready to be a mother. I can see it—you are ready. Nothing in your past can hold you back from having a child. You deserve this! You are worthy of this! There is nothing to fear when it comes to becoming a mother. You can do this. Millions of women from various backgrounds, life experiences and families do this. So can you. You do not need to be perfect to be a good mother. Go ahead, let yourself have this. You deserve a baby.

Love,

_____

For more letters to send yourself, Dancing Your Way to Fertility can be purchased at Amazon.com or at www.dancingyourwaytofertility.com.

www.ingramcontent.com/pod-product-compliance
Lightning Source LLC
Chambersburg PA
CBHW081653270326
41933CB00017B/3155